The Story of
Iodine Deficiency

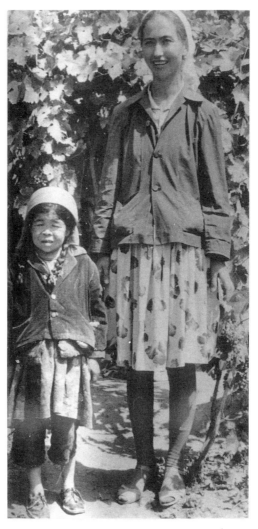

Left: A myxoedematous cretin from Sinjiang, China who is also deaf mute. This condition is completely preventable. Right: The barefoot doctor of her village. Both are about 35 years of age. (Photograph kindly made available by Professor T. Ma of Tianjin, People's Republic of China.)

The Story of Iodine Deficiency

An International Challenge in Nutrition

BASIL S. HETZEL

Executive Director
International Council for Control of
Iodine Deficiency Disorders

OXFORD NEW YORK TOKYO
OXFORD UNIVERSITY PRESS
1989

Oxford University Press, Walton Street, Oxford OX2 6DP

Oxford   New York   Toronto
Delhi   Bombay   Calcutta   Madras   Karachi
Petaling Jaya   Singapore   Hong Kong   Tokyo
Nairobi   Dar es Salaam   Cape Town
Melbourne   Auckland

and associated companies in
Berlin   Ibadan

Oxford is a trade mark of Oxford University Press

Published in the United States
by Oxford University Press, New York

British Library Cataloguing in Publication Data

Hetzel, Basil S. (Basil Stuart), 1922–
The story of iodine deficiency: an international challenge in nutrition.
1. Man. Diseases. Role of iodine deficiency
I. Title
616.3'96

ISBN 0-19-261669-2
ISBN 0-19-261866-0 (Pbk)

Library of Congress Cataloging in Publication Data

Hetzel, Basil S., 1922–
The story of iodine deficiency.
Includes index.
1. Iodine deficiency diseases—Prevention.   I. Title.
[DNLM: 1. Iodine—deficiency.   2. Nutrition Disorders—
prevention & control.   QV 283 H591s]
RA645.I55H47   1989   616.3'9   88-31253

ISBN 0-19-261669-2
ISBN 0-19-261866-0 (Pbk)

Set by Colset Private Limited, Singapore
Printed in Great Britain by
St Edmundsbury Press,
Bury St Edmunds, Suffolk

Preface

Today we have the necessary knowledge to correct iodine deficiency for the nearly 1 billion people at risk. This book presents this knowledge in the belief that many, once informed, will wish to see it applied without further delay. I hope that they will be willing to take steps to achieve that end through the national and international discussion that is required for the necessary political decisions.

There is a great opportunity now for an application of science and technology with incalculable benefits to human well-being for many hundreds of millions living in an iodine deficient environment all over the world.

The author is indebted to many friends and colleagues throughout the world who share his interest in the prevention and control of iodine deficiency disorders (IDD). This book presents the knowledge that this whole group has acquired over the past 25 years that is now ready for application. Most of these colleagues are members of the recently established International Council for Control of Iodine Deficiency Disorders (ICCIDD)—a body that has been set up to bridge the wide knowledge–application gap that exists about IDD and its control.

Dr John Stanbury, Chairman of the ICCIDD, Dr V. Ramalingaswami, Vice Chairman of the ICCIDD, and Dr John Dunn, Secretary of the ICCIDD and Editor of the *IDD Newsletter*, are particularly able, congenial, and willing colleagues in the work of the ICCIDD.

We are particularly appreciative of the strong support that has been provided by Drs E. DeMaeyer, Kenneth Bailey and Graeme Clugston of WHO, Mr David Haxton, Mr Rolf Carriere, and Dr Peter Greaves of UNICEF.

To many other colleagues in Australia and overseas, I am also indebted.

The production costs of this book have been subsidized by a grant from the International Council for the Control of Iodine Deficiency Disorders.

Finally, the staunch support of my wife, Anne, and my secretary, Lyn Giehl, are also acknowledged with gratitude and thanks.

Adelaide, Australia　　　　　　　　　　　　　　　　B.S.H.
June 1988

'Iodine deficiency is so easy to prevent that it is a crime to let a single child be born mentally handicapped for that reason'

LABOUISSE (UNICEF) 1978

Contents

Introduction

Iodine deficiency is a risk factor for the growth and development of up to 800 million people living in iodine deficient environments throughout the world. The effects on growth and development, called the iodine deficiency disorders (IDD), comprise goitre, still-births and miscarriages, neonatal and juvenile thyroid deficiency, dwarfism, mental defects, deaf mutism, and spastic weakness and paralysis, as well as lesser degrees of loss of physical and mental function. All these effects are due to inadequate thyroid hormone production because iodine is an essential constituent of the thyroid hormone.

In the West, IDD has been largely eliminated by the addition of iodine to the diet through iodized salt or through changes in food distribution and technology. IDD still persists in certain areas of Europe where these dietary changes have not occurred.

In the Third World, IDD is a major problem in many countries with large populations, such as China, India, Indonesia, Nigeria, and Zaire. In these and other Third World countries, IDD is a significant barrier to social and economic progress which can be removed by correction of the deficiency.

This book shows that elimination of iodine deficiency is feasible within the next decade, only requiring a modest financial and technical effort from the West. Part I reviews IDD in man and animals. Part II discusses the control of iodine deficiency disorders through iodine supplementation, and considers action at the national and international level. Part III presents a global review of the status of IDD control. There is a brief conclusion on the way forward to successful control programmes.

Glossary

colloid	constituent of the thyroid gland in which thyroid hormone storage takes place
creatinine	a product of metabolism in muscle which is excreted in the urine at about the same level from day to day
CSIRO	Commonwealth Scientific and Industrial Research Organization, Australia
diplegia	a state of paralysis affecting the legs
epiphyses	the growing end of bones
Ethiodol	another name for Lipiodol (see below)
goitrogens	substances in the diet which produce goitre due to action on the thyroid gland in blocking thyroid hormone synthesis or increasing kidney excretion of iodide. Their effect can usually be overcome by increasing iodine intake
hippocampus	part of the brain concerned with emotion
hyperplasia	increased number of cells due to stimulation
hyperthyroidism	a condition due to elevated levels of thyroid hormones which produce a rapid heart rate and other features of a nervous state (trembling, excessive sweating, irritability, and loss of weight)
hypothyroidism	the result of a lowered level of circulating thyroid hormone with slowing of mental and physical functions
iodate	e.g. potassium iodate (KIO_3) an iodine containing salt, more stable than potassium iodide in the moist tropics

iodide	iodine in chemically bound form usually with sodium or potassium as a salt
iodism	sensitivity to iodine, indicated by a skin rash
iodophors	iodine-containing antiseptics used in the dairy industry
leucine	an amino-acid which is a constituent of proteins
linoleic acid	a polyunsaturated fatty acid with 18 carbon atoms and two double bonds, which is a major constituent of vegetable oils, especially sunflower or safflower oils
Lipiodol	radio-opaque dye used in radiology for many years
myxoedema	the result of severe hypothyroidism, when the skin and subcutaneous tissue thicken because of accumulation of mucin
QRS	the major electrical impulse in the heart that causes the heartbeat and is recorded in an electrocardiogram
radio-opaque	opaque or dense to X-rays
thiocyanate	substance produced in the liver by metabolism of cyanide from eating cassava
thyroxine (T_4)	thyroid hormone which contains four atoms of iodine; known chemically as tetraiodothyronine
triiodothyronine (T_3)	thyroid hormone containing three atoms of iodine
TSH	thyroid-stimulating hormone which comes from the pituary gland at the base of the brain

PART I
Understanding iodine deficiency

1

The history of goitre and cretinism

The story of iodine deficiency begins with a review of the history of goitre and cretinism. These obvious abnormalities of the human body and human behaviour, in the form of a lump in the neck and mental deficiency, have aroused comment and speculation over the whole of recorded history. Because the people of each period interpreted the problem according to cultural context, this account provides a fascinating example of the continuous grappling of the human mind with an unusual natural phenomenon.

The first records of goitre and cretinism date back to the ancient civilizations, the Chinese and Hindu cultures, and then to Greece and Rome. In the Middle Ages, goitrous cretins appeared in the pictoral art, often as angels or demons. The first detailed descriptions of these subjects occurred in the Renaissance. The paintings of the Madonnas in Italy so commonly showed goitre that the condition must have been regarded as virtually normal. In the 17th and 18th centuries, scientific studies multiplied, and the first recorded mention of the word 'cretin' appeared in Diderot's *Encyclopédie* in 1754. The 19th century marked the beginning of serious attempts to control the problem; however, not until the latter half of the 20th century have we acquired the necessary knowledge for effective prevention and control.

In the following account I have made extensive reference to two previous comprehensive reviews, both published in the WHO monograph in 1960 (Kelly and Snedden 1960; Langer 1960). I have also referred to the excellent review of König (1981) on the history of cretinism. These reviews provide a comprehensive series of original references to which the reader is referred for follow up as desired.

The ancient civilizations

One of the oldest references to goitre is attributed to the legendary Chinese Shen-Nung Emperor (2838–2698 BC) who, in his book

Pen-Ts'ao Tsing (*A treatise on herbs and roots*) is said to have mentioned the seaweed Sargasso as an effective remedy for goitre. A little later, 2697–2597 BC, two types of neck tumours were recognized, those caused by an accumulation of air (possibly tumours) and those brought about by an accumulation of blood (possibly inflammatory swellings). Goitre was also mentioned in the book from the period 770–220 BC, *Shan Khai Tsing* (*A treatise on waters and dry lands*), which attributed the disease to the poor quality of the water. Other references during the Han dynasty (206 BC–AD 220 and the Wei dynasty (AD 200–264) attributed deep emotions and 'certain conditions of life in the mountain regions' as causes of goitre. The treatment of goitre with Sargasso and another seaweed *Laminaria japonica tresch*, was mentioned by the famous Chinese medical writer Ge-Khun who lived between AD 317 and 419. The Chinese even used animal thyroid in the treatment of goitre: the use of deer thyroid was mentioned in the book by Shen Shi-Fan (AD 420–501). Animal thyroid continued to be used in China, and the eminent Chinese physician Li Shi-Chen (Ming dynasty 1552–1578) discussed preparations of pig and deer thyroid in the well known herbal *Pen-T'sao Kang-Mu*.

The continued use of seaweed and animal thyroid over so many hundreds of years suggests that there was certainly some benefit derived from these measures in the treatment of goitre.

In the ancient Hindu literature, incantations against goitre are found in the Atharva-Veda dating from around 2000 BC.

Tumours of the neck were also known in Ancient Egypt, where they were treated surgically according to the Ebers papyrus (c. 1500 BC).

The oldest known representation of goitre is in the Buddha frieze of Gandhara, now in Pakistan (2nd/3rd century AD). The frieze (Fig. 1.1) shows Buddha beset on all sides with animals and human beings who seek to disturb his meditation. Among these figures is a man with a large goitre. He is carrying a drum which the man behind him is beating with a crook. His facial expression suggests idiocy, and we may even speculate that he is deaf in view of the close proximity of the drum to his ears. This 'cretin' is representative of many goitrous individuals that are still to be seen in Northern Pakistan today (Blumberg and Baruch 1964).

Professor F. Merke of Basle, in his remarkable *History and iconography of endemic goitre and cretinism* (1984) points out that

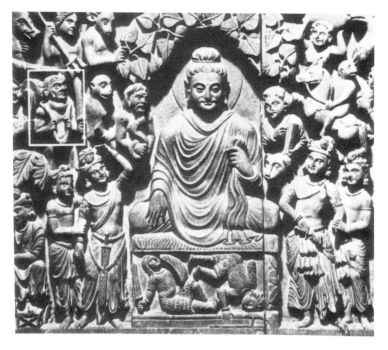

Fig. 1.1. A Buddha freize from Gandhara 2nd/3rd century. Among the disturbers of the peace can be seen (top left) a man with a large goitre, a stupid expression, and a drum on his back. (After Blumberg 1964 and Merke 1984, with permission).

this particular frieze demonstrates Graeco–Roman influences on Oriental art. This began with the Indian campaigns of Alexander the Great in which he was accompanied not only by soldiers, but also by scholars and artists. Some 500 years later Roman elements were incorporated in the art of the region. In the frieze, Buddha is given human form and wears a Roman toga!

Several Roman authors commented on the prevalence of goitre in the Alps. The poet Juvenal (1st century A D) asked, 'Who wonders at a swelling of the neck in the Alps?' ('Quis turindum guttur miratus in Alpibus?'). The architect Vitruvius (1st century B C) stated that the Aqui in Italy and the Medulli in the Alps got a swelling of the neck from their drinking water. Pliny the Elder (1st century A D) agreed about the importance of drinking water in causing a swelling of the throat. Caesar apparently noticed swollen necks among the Gauls during the course of his military campaigns.

The 'father of medicine', Hippocrates of the Greek island of Cos, regarded poor drinking water as a cause of goitre, as revealed in the famous volume, *Air, water and places*. Celsus (25 BC–AD 45) described a fleshy tumour of the neck which he incised, to find it contained honey-like substances even with small bones and hairs—this was probably a long standing goitre. It was subsequently deduced by the great physician Galen (AD 132–200) that the glands of the neck, including the thyroid, had the function of secreting a fluid into the larynx and the pharynx. These views continued to be accepted for many centuries and were certainly held by the great physicians Malipighi in Italy (1628–1694) and Boerhaave in Holland (1668–1738).

The Middle Ages

It is of great interest to note the attention given to goitre in paintings and sculptures in the Middle Ages. This has been a subject of particular interest to the late Professor F. Merke of Basle (1984) who carried out investigations over many years. He unearthed the following interesting examples from manuscripts and churches.

The earliest illustration of goitre and cretinism was found in the Austrian National Library in Vienna in the *Reuner Musterbuch* dating from 1215, a book coming from the Cistercian Abbey in Reun near Graz in Styria, Austria, where goitre has been highly endemic until recent times. The picture (Fig. 1.2) shows a figure with three large goitres and a stupid facial expression brandishing a fool's staff in one hand, and reaching up with the other towards a toad. This must be a goitrous cretin—it was common to depict a fool as grasping a cudgel. The significance of the toad may be related to the popular use of live or dismembered frogs for the treatment of goitre. As Merke points out, this picture of the Reun cretin predates by some 300 years the recognition of the relation between goitre and cretinism by Paracelsus (1493–1541).

In the 13th century, there were two encyclopaedias which recorded fables of human monsters from Greek and Indian mythology. Some descriptions of giant goitres were also included based on observations *'in extrerius Burgundiae circa Alpes'*. One of the encylopaedists, Jacques de Vitiga was much travelled, had been

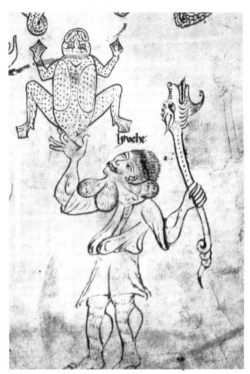

Fig. 1.2. 'The Reun cretin' from the Reun Model Book *Reuner Musterbruch* produced by the Cistercian Abbey at Reun (near Graz) Austria and dating from 1215. This model book covers everything that an educated 'clericus' of the 13th century had to know. The cretin has a large trilobed goitre with the third lobe strung over the left shoulder. His right hand clutches at a frog (possibly for healing) and his left hand holds the 'fool's sceptre' in order to make the mental deficiency clear (after Merke 1984, with permission).

involved with the Cossacks, and must have passed through the Alpine passes several times, and so had the opportunity to see goitrous and cretin subjects (König 1981).

In the middle of the 14th century another figure appeared in the psalter of St. Lambrecht ascribed to the year 1346. The figure has a vacant pasty face with an infantile expression; in his left hand he holds a fool's staff with a pig's bladder attached to the top: a symbol of the fool like the cudgel in the previous picture. His right hand holds the very large twin-lobed goitre. St. Lambrecht is a village in Carinthia, Austria, which like Styria has had widespread goitre and cretinism for centuries.

These sufferers were in fact given special recognition in the medieval world, where they were often regarded as angels or innocents with magical powers (Merke 1984). Clearly the medieval world could not ignore these individuals, but did its best to fit them into the prevailing religious culture.

The origin of the term 'cretin' was discussed by De Quervain and Wegelin (1936). They considered the most likely origin to be 'Christianus' or 'Crestin' in the south-eastern French dialect, referring to a 'bon chretien' because of the innocence of these subjects.

In the last quarter of the 15th century, the Swiss Chronicles included illustrations of goitrous Bernese and Valaisian warriors in the description of their raids on one another. One illustration (Fig. 1.3) shows a Bernese warrior slitting the goitres of the unfortunate Valaisians, indicating a significant disadvantage to the goitrous subject!

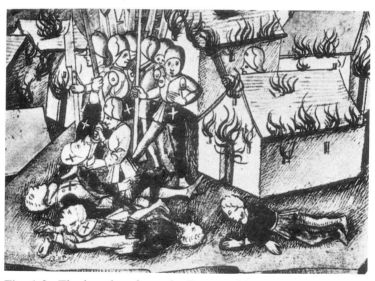

Fig. 1.3. The invaders from the Bernese Oberland set fire to Sion and massacre the Valaisians by running swords through their goitres. (*T. Schachtlan Chronicle* after Merke 1984, with permission.)

Surgical operations were described from the early medical schools at Salerno (1170), Montpellier (1240), and Padua (1252). Sea sponges were also used and continued to be recommended into the 19th century. Various beliefs arose about the causes of goitre: that it arose from strenuous work, or frequent fits of coughing, and that it occurred in women after a difficult labour—which is the origin of the custom of tying a lace around the neck during labour. The moon was also thought to be involved (Langer 1960).

Marco Polo saw goitres in Russian Central Asia (formerly Turkestan) when on his famous travels from Venice to the court of the Grand Khan of China in 1275. This region is immediately west of the Chinese province of Sinjiang where I saw severe goitre and cretinism in 1982.

The Renaissance

Felix Platter (1536–1614) of Basle vividly described goitre and cretinism following his visit to the Valais with his father in 1562. His classic description reads:

In Bremis, a village of the Valais, as I have seen myself, and in the Valley of Carinthia called Binthzgerthal [today the Pinzgau], it is usual that many infants suffer from innate folly [simplemindedness]. Besides, the head is sometimes misshapen: the tongue is huge and swollen; they are dumb; the throat is often goiterous. Thus, they present an ugly sight; and sitting in the streets and looking into the sun, and putting little sticks in between their fingers, twisting their bodies in various ways, with their mouths agape they provoke passers by to laughter and astonishment.

(Langer 1960.)

Joseph Simmler (1530–1576) of Zurich described cretins in the canton of Valais, while the Dutch physician Pieter van Foreest (died 1597) noted the many cretins in the province of Valtellina on the Italian side of the Swiss border (König 1981).

A study of goitre in 16th century art has been made by Hunziger (1935). Goitre can be readily observed in the madonnas of Renaissance masters such as Van Eyck and Lucas Van der Leyden. These madonnas may be observed today in the Sienese and Vatican galleries (Fig. 1.4). That Mary was portrayed with this feature, and that she was portrayed thus by more than one artist, suggests that goitre was accepted as normal and certainly not as a stigma. Indeed, it was regarded as a sign of a Visitation of God. Goitre may also be seen in

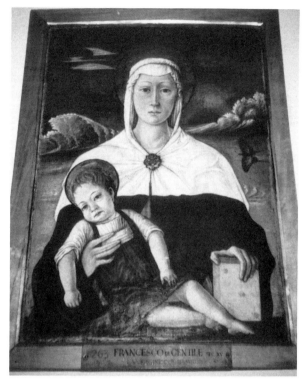

Fig. 1.4. Madonna and child by Francesco di Gentili, 15th century. The madonna has a goitre and her child looks hypothyroid (from Vatican Museum, Rome).

the later paintings of Rubens, Weyden, and Durer.

There were, however, many views about goitre. It was believed to be cured by the touch of a king. In France, Henry IV, according to his personal physician, caused 1500 goitres to regress by touching the patient and using the formula, 'Le Roi te touche et Dieu te Guerit.' This was practised by many English Kings, including Charles II who is alleged to have touched 9200 sufferers of the King's Evil or scrofula, with which goitre was often confused. According to newspaper reports, Queen Anne on 20th March 1710, revived the ancient custom of curing goitre by the laying on of hands.

As already mentioned, Paracelsus recognized the association of goitre and cretinism and also attributed the disease to a deficiency of minerals in drinking water, which contrasts the scientific approach with the magic of the king's touch.

The seventeenth century

The study of human anatomy prospered following the great pioneering work of Andreas Vesalius, Realdus Colombus, Fabricius, and Eustachius in the 16th century. All of these great anatomists noted the thyroid gland, which was called the 'glandulus laryngis' by Vesalius. Fabricius recognized the connection between the glandulus laryngis and goitre.

It was the Englishman, Thomas Wharton (1614–1673) whose work *Adenography or a description of the glands of the entire body*, published in London in 1656, contained the first description of the gland:

It contributes much to the rotundity and beauty of the neck, filling up the vacant spaces round the larynx, and making its protuberant parts almost to subside and become smooth, particularly in females, to whom for this reason a larger gland has been assigned, which renders their necks more even and beautiful.

However, the function of the thyroid was not understood—it was usually regarded as secretory fluid to 'humidify' the walls of the larynx, the pharynx, and the trachea. The function of the thyroid was not in fact unravelled until the latter part of the 19th century when it was recognized to have an 'internal' secretion in the form of the thyroid hormone, and not an external one.

The eighteenth century

In the 18th century there was a great escalation in scientific observations and reports of these observations. These were collected in Diderot's *Encylopedie on dictionnaire raisonne des sciences* published in 1754. The term 'cretin' probably appeared in print for the first time in 1754 in an article by Diderot's co-editor, d'Alembert. The definition of a cretin given was, 'an imbecile who is deaf and dumb with a goitre hanging down to the waist'. The endemic nature of goitre led to the use of the term 'endemic cretinism'. Although a goitre was usually present, this was not always the case (see Chapter 3).

There were many reports published. Of special interest is that of B.E. Fodére (1764–1836), a physician who was born in the Savoie–Val d'Aoste. His book, *Traite du goitre et du crétinisme*, was published several times in French and German at the turn of the century. A portrait of a cretin subject from Martigny in the Valais is shown in Figure 1.5 and gives some idea of the clinical phenomenon that these authors were observing and writing about.

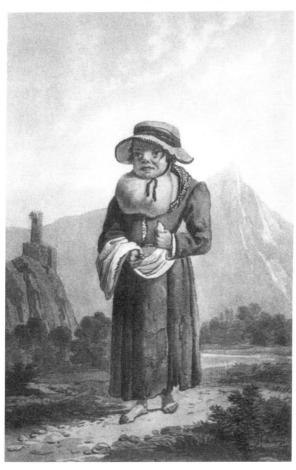

Fig. 1.5. Goitrous cretin woman from Martigny, Valais. Aquarelle painted by Almeraz in 1820. (After Merke 1984, with permission).

The nineteenth century

An escalation of interest and concern about the possibility of controlling this problem occurred at the beginning of the 19th century. Napoleon ordered a systematic investigation of goitre because of the large numbers of young men from certain regions who were rejected as unfit for military duties. He probably had seen something of the problem on his march into Italy through the Valais.

In a book published in 1844 by Rosch and Maffei it was concluded that there was no uniform clinical manifestation of a cretin, but there was in fact a wide spectrum of clinical symptomatology. The authors also recorded the remarkable observations of a family living in a certain house where the children were cretinous or died very young. When, however, the family was living elsewhere before and after the birth of the cretins, several normal children were born.

In 1848, a special commission was appointed by King Carlo Alberto of Sardinia to study the extent of goitre throughout his Kingdom, which at that time included the provinces of Savoy, Nice, Piedmont, Genoa, and the Island of Sardinia, and to recommend the means of controlling it. Ten years later the Commission submitted its report, which recorded that 370 403 persons in France above the age of 20 had goitre and that in addition there were approximately 120 000 cretins and idiots (the total population of France at that time was about 36 million).

What about control of this problem? At this time there was great diversity in opinion on the causes of goitre. In 1867 Saint-Lager listed 43 different views on the causes of goitre expressed by 378 authors. Nineteen of these views attributed the disease to various properties of water (its origin, or its deficiency or excess of certain minerals); eleven thought the atmosphere was important (humidity, temperature, chemical composition, and lack of sunshine); six pointed to faulty nutrition, poverty, and unsanitary living conditions; and the remaining seven blamed other factors such as alcoholism and consanguinity in marriage. The relationship between iodine and goitre was probably suspected soon after. However it was not until 1896 that the presence of iodine in the thyroid was first demonstrated by Baumann.

Iodine was isolated from the ashes of the seaweed *Fucus vesicularis* by Courtois in France in 1813. Coindet (1774–1848) in 1820 recommended iodine preparations for the treatment of goitre, and on 25 July 1820 made a report in a lecture to the Swiss Society of Natural Sciences in Geneva. However, soon afterwards there was marked opposition because of the occurrence of symptoms of toxicity (heart disorder, wasting, and, disturbed menstruation) which we now know was due to excessive thyroid secretion (iodine-induced hyperthyroidism, see Chapter 7).

Coindet (1820) had been very careful in the dosage he had used and had not had any such toxic effects in 150 patients he had treated. Jean Louis Prévost (1790–1850) observed that very low doses (0.9–2.0 mg) were sufficient to cause some regression of goitre, from which he deduced that goitre might be caused by a deficiency of iodine or bromine in water, and that the condition might be prevented by giving iodine. In 1846 with an Italian colleague, A. C. Maffoni, Prévost put forward for the first time the theory that goitre was due to iodine deficiency (Prévost and Maffoni 1846).

The iodization of salt was first suggested by Boussingault, who lived for many years in Colombia, South America. He learnt that the local people benefited from salt obtained from an abandoned mine in Guaca, Antioquia. In 1825 Boussingault analysed this salt and found large quantities of iodine, and subsequently suggested in 1833 that iodized salt be used for the prevention of goitre.

The first controlled experiment was carried out in France. Goitrous families received salt fortified with 0.1–0.5 g of potassium iodide per kilogram of salt. Again symptoms of an excess thyroid secretion occurred due to the high dosage, and the treatment fell again into disrepute.

The twentieth century

Present-day practice in the prevention and control of goitre is based on the work of David Marine, who in 1915 declared that 'endemic goitre is the easiest known disease to prevent'. In the same year Hunziger proposed that iodized salt be used for goitre control in Switzerland.

The first large-scale trials with iodine were carried out over the period 1916–20 by Marine and Kimball (1922) in Akron, Ohio, USA. About 5000 girls between 11 and 18 years of age took part in this experiment. Of these, 2190 were given a daily dose of 0.2 g of sodium iodide in water for ten days in the spring and ten days in the autumn, making a total dose of 4.0 g over the year. The remaining 2305 girls acted as controls. The results are summarized in Table 1.1. Two facts stand out from these data:

1. In the group receiving sodium iodide, out of 908 girls with a normal thyroid prior to treatment, only 2, i.e. 0.2 per cent developed goitre, whereas among the 1257 girls of the control group with previously normal thyroid, goitre appeared in 347, or 27.6 per cent.

2. In the treated group, 773 out of 1282 girls with goitre, i.e. 60.4 per cent, showed a considerable decrease in the size of the thyroid, while in the control group spontaneous regression of the goitre occurred only in 145 out of 1048 girls, i.e. 13.8 per cent.

Both the prophylactic and the therapeutic effects were thus impressive. Iodism (sensitivity to iodine indicated by a skin rash) was very rare (only 11 cases) in spite of the extremely large doses of iodine; and the symptoms disappeared within a few days of stopping the administration of sodium iodide.

Table 1.1 *Results of iodine prophylaxis in Akron, Ohio, USA, from 1917–1919**

Size of the thyroid	With iodine		Without iodine	
	No.	%	No.	%
Normal:				
Unchanged	906	99.8	910	72.4
Increased	2	0.2	347	27.6
Slightly enlarged:				
Unchanged	477	41.9	698	72.8
Increased	3	0.3	127	13.3
Decreased	659	57.8	134	13.9
Moderately enlarged:				
Unchanged	29	20.3	57	64.0
Increased	—	—	21	23.6
Decreased	114	79.7	11	12.4
Total	2190	100.0	2305	100.0

* After Marine and Kimball by kind permission of the editors of the *American Journal of the Medical Sciences* (1922), cited by Kelly and Snedden (1960).

Mass prophylaxis of goitre with iodized salt was first introduced on a community scale in Michigan in 1924 (Kimball 1937). Goitre surveys in schoolchildren and iodine analyses of the drinking-water were first carried out in 4 representative counties, namely Houghton, Wexford, Midland, and McComb. The average goitre rate among the 65 537 schoolchildren examined was 38.6 per cent. Table salt containing 1 part in 5000 of potassium iodide was then introduced, and by 1929 the rate had fallen to 9 per cent. The follow-up survey conducted by Brush and Altland in 1951 on 53 785 school-children in the same counties gave a goitre rate of only 1.4 per cent. It was also reported that in 7 large hospitals in Michigan, thyroid-ectomies accounted for only 1 per cent of all operations in 1950 compared with 3.2 per cent in 1939. No toxic symptoms of iodide prophylaxis were observed.

The impact of iodized salt in the control of goitre is vividly illustrated by events in Switzerland. The prevalence of goitre and cretinism was very great throughout the whole country, situated as it is in the elevated region of the European Alps. The burden of cretinism was a heavy charge on public funds: in 1923 the Canton of Berne alone with a population of little more than 700 000 had to hospitalize 700 cretins incapable of self-care. However, following the introduction of iodized salt, goitre incidence fell steeply. Later, deaf and dumb institutions were closed or diverted for other purposes. Observations of army recruits showed definite evidence of this trend (Table 1.2). Between the years 1925 and 1947 the number of exemp-

Table 1.2 *Incidence of goitre among army recruits in Switzerland*

Year	Number of men examined	Number of men exempt on account of goitre	Number of goitres per 1000
1900	26 285	2451	93.2
1905	26 448	3093	116.9
1914–18	151 106	3403	22.5
1921	32 838	1817	55.3
1925	39 681	1229	30.9
1935	29 627	338	11.4
1939–45	228 101	340	1.5
1945	31 654	21	0.6
1947	31 366	23	0.7

From Schamb (1949), by permission. Cited by Kelly and Snedden (1960).

Table 1.3 *Incidence of goitre among schoolchildren in the canton of Valais*

Period	Normal thyroids (%)	Palpable thyroids (%)	Enlarged neck (%)	Pronounced goitres (%)
1920 (Before introduction of iodized salt)	28.8	54.3	14.9	2.0
1934 (Ten years after introduction of iodized salt in 1924)	70.5	27.3	2.1	0.15

From Bayard (1937), by permission. Cited by Kelly and Snedden (1960).

tions for military service fell from 31 to less than 1 per thousand.

A big decline in goitre was also seen among schoolchildren in the canton of Valais, which had a particularly severe problem (see Table 1.3).

In Switzerland the use of iodized salt was controlled at canton level and not federal level, so that there was a considerable difference in the timing and in the quantity sold. This is reflected in the goitre statistics; there was a reduction in goitre in the conscripts much earlier from those cantons which introduced prophylaxis in 1922, 1923, and 1924, than from those which did not introduce it until 1929 or 1930.

In Austria, as in Switzerland, the prevalence of goitre was high throughout the country. There was an increase in prevalence after each of the World Wars, particularly evident in the newborn. Iodine was given from the third day of life to infants with neonatal goitre. However, it was also reported that administration of potassium iodide to pregnant women before the fourth month reduced the goitre rate in the newborn from 47 per cent to about 5 per cent in the space of two years.

In Italy, goitre and cretinism still occurs to a varying degree throughout the whole of the northern Alpine region, including Piedmont, Lombardy, and Trentino, to Venezia in the east. The condition also occurs in the plains north and south of the River Po, in the Apennines north of Genoa, in Tuscany, and in many other areas including Sicily, reflecting the generally hilly nature of the terrain throughout Italy.

In the Valtellina valley in the North, which follows the River Adda into Lake Como, goitre prophylaxis with iodized salt had by 1938 been in vogue for about 14 years with good results. There had been a fall in goitre rate from 57 per cent to 1.4 per cent. There was improved mental alertness in children with a lowering of infant mortality.

In Northern Italy high rates of goitre with persistent cretinism have been reported from the Upper Isarco Valley in the Trentino Upper Adige area (Platzer *et al.* 1975). There was previously a high rejection rate of recruits in the whole province of Bolzano: 9.5 per cent in 1907, 2.63 per cent in 1916 and 1.49 per cent in 1923, compared to mean values of 0.37 per cent, 0.15 per cent, and 0.45 per cent for Italy as a whole. There was also a higher rate of death from cancer of the thyroid—another indication of iodine deficiency—11.5 per 1000 cancer deaths in Upper Adige compared to 4.6 per 1000 for Italy as a whole. Goitre rates ranging from 29–84 per cent (mean 48.6 per cent) were found in schoolchildren, with low urinary iodine (mean 25 μg/g creatinine in 253 children). Low dietary iodine was confirmed by measurements on the available foods compared to those in the cities of Turin and Piedmont. Endemic cretins were seen in the age range 31–77, of whom four were deaf mute.

However, there has been a general decline in goitre and cretinism in the Alpine area. This has occurred following the introduction of iodized salt in Switzerland, but has also occurred in some cantons where iodized salt has not been introduced. In Piedmont, Italy this decline has been particularly well-documented by Dr Costa and his colleagues at the Institute of Endocrine and Metabolic Diseases, Maruiziano Hospital, Turin. A downward trend had become apparent as early as the end of the 18th century and was noted by the Sardinia Commission in Piedmont in 1848. A further decline was apparent by the beginning of the 20th century. In 1964 Costa and his colleagues estimated the prevalence of cretinism to be in the region of 0.1 per 1000 compared with 1.53 per thousand in 1881. Overall the number of registered deaf mutes was estimated to be 0.79 per 1000 in Piedmont reaching 2.85 in the endemic goitre areas where cretinism is more common. (Costa *et al.* 1964)

The important feature noted in Piedmont was that a decline in cretinism had occurred not only in the upper Aosta Valley where iodine prophylaxis was carried out, but also in other regions (Cuneo and Maritime Alps) where no iodine prophylaxis had been instituted. In other words, the same situation had occurred as in Switzerland. Similarly, in Yugoslavia, Ramzin *et al.* (1968) had noted a fall in cretinism from 13 per cent before 1930 to 7 per cent following economic development, and then finally a disappearance following the introduction of iodine prophylaxis in 1954.

The question raised, therefore, was whether iodine deficiency was indeed the significant factor in the causation of endemic cretinism. This was a subject of much controversy. It led to the controlled trial in Papua New Guinea in 1966, which will be described in Chapter 4. The results of this trial supported by other observations of the effect of iodine prophylaxis have established iodine deficiency during pregnancy as the major cause of cretinism. The disappearance of cretinism can be attributed to an increase in iodine intake as a result of the diversification of the diet that accompanies economic development. The persistence of goitre and cretinism in various remote areas such as Sicily can be attributed to the persistence of iodine deficiency because economic development has not occurred. These communities have continued to rely mainly on local food, particularly cereals, in the local iodine deficient soil usually in mountains or hilly areas.

At this stage, we can conclude from our historical review that goitre and cretinism have aroused much speculation and comment throughout human history. However, it is only in the latter part of the 20th century that we have acquired the necessary knowledge for successful prevention and control of the problem. It remains for the present generation to bring about the necessary application of this knowledge to eradicate an ancient scourge of mankind. The questions of prevention and control are fully discussed in Parts II and III. The next five chapters of this book describe the development of knowledge since 1950 of the effects of iodine deficiency.

Bibliography and further reading

Baumann, E. (1895). *Hoppe-Seyl. Z. physiol. Chem.* **21**, 319.

Blumberg, B. and Baruch, S. (1964). Goiter in Ghandara. A representation in a second to third century frieze. *Journal of the American Medical Association* **199**.

Brush, B.E. and Altland, J.K. (1952). *Journal of Clinical Endocrinology,* **12**, 1380.

Coindet, J.F. (1820). *Bibl. universelle Sci. Arts Geneve* **14**, 190.

Costa, A., Cottino, F., Mortara, M., and Vogliazzao, V. (1964). Endemic cretinism in Piedmont. *Panminerva Medica* **6**, 250–9.

Courtois, M.B. (1813). *Ann. Chim. Paris* **88**, 304.

De Quervain, F., and Wegelin, C. (1936). Der endemische Kretinismus, Berlin and Vienna.

Fodére, M. (1792). Assai sur le goitre et le crétiniage. De l'Impremiur Royale.

Hunziger, H. (1935). *Schweiz. Med. Wschr.* **65**, 13.

Kelly, F.C. and Snedden, W.W. (1960). The prevalence and geographical distribution of endemic goitre. In *Endemic goitre*, pp. 27–234. World Health Organization, Geneva.

Kimball, O.P. (1937). *Journal of the American Medical Association* **198**, 860.

König, P. (1981) 'Myxedematous' and 'nervous cretinism': a historical review. In *Fetal brain disorders* (eds. B.S. Hetzel and R.M. Smith), pp. 229–42. Elsevier, Amsterdam.

Langer, P. (1960). The history of goitre. In *Endemic goitre*, pp. 9–25. World Health Organization, Geneva.

Marine, D. (1914). *Journal of Experimental Medicine* **19**, 70.

Marine, D., and Kimball, O.P. (1922). The prevention of simple goitre. *American Journal of Medical Sciences* **163**, 634.

Merke, F. (1984). *The history and iconography of endemic goitre and cretinism.* MTP Press, Lancaster (originally published by Hans Huber, Berne, in 1971).

2

The biology of iodine

Iodine is an essential element for normal growth and development in animals and man. It occurs in the human body in only small amounts (15–20 mg) and the essential requirement for normal growth is only 100–150 μg per day (0.1–0.15 mg). Because of this, iodine is referred to as a 'trace element'. It has a relatively high atomic weight (127) which is more than twice that of the next heaviest element in the body, cobalt, which has an atomic weight of 60. Most of the common organic elements are much smaller—carbon (12), hydrogen (11), and oxygen (16).

The special biological importance of iodine arises from the fact that it is a constituent of the thyroid hormones thyroxine 3,5,3′5′—tetraiodothyronine (T_4) and 3,5,3′—triiodothyronine (T_3) (Fig. 2.1).

TETRAIODOTHYRONINE (THYROXINE)

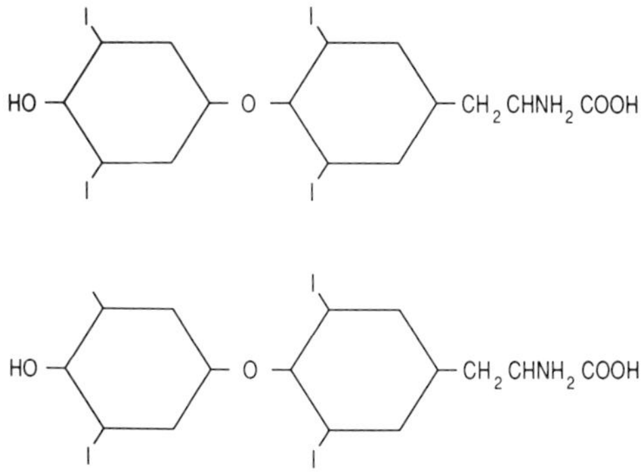

TRIIODOTHYRONINE

Fig. 2.1. Chemical formulae of thyroxine, or tetraiodothyronine (T_4), and triiodothyronine (T_3).

The iodine cycle in nature

There is a cycle of iodine in nature. Most iodine resides in the ocean. It was present during the primordial development of the earth, but large amounts were leached from the surface soil by glaciation, snow, and rain, and were carried by wind, rivers, and floods into the sea. Iodine occurs in the deeper layers of the soil and is found in oil-well effluents. Water from deep wells can provide a major source of iodine. In general, the older an exposed soil surface the more likely it is to be leached of iodine. The most likely areas to be leached are mountainous areas. The most severely deficient are the Himalayas, the Andes, the European Alps, and the vast mountains of China. But iodine deficiency is likely to occur in all elevated regions subject to higher rainfall, with run-off into rivers (Fig. 2.2).

Glaciation is a major cause of iodine loss from the soil in mountainous regions. A study of this relationship has been made in

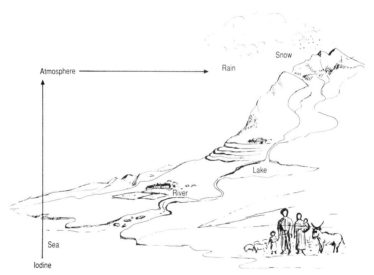

Fig. 2.2. The iodine cycle in nature. The atmosphere absorbs iodine from the sea which then returns through the rain and snow to the mountainous regions. It is then carried by rivers to the lower hills and plains, eventually returning to the sea. High rainfall, snow, and flooding increase the loss of soil iodine which has often been already denuded by past glaciation. This causes the low iodine content of food for man and animals.

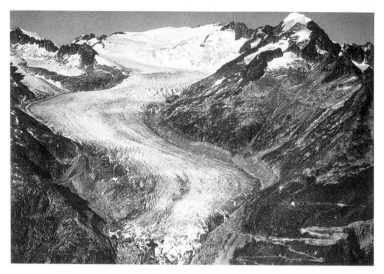

Fig. 2.3. The Rhone glacier is responsible for the loss of iodine from the soil of the Valais and adjacent areas in Switzerland. (From A. Kiener.)

Switzerland (Fig. 2.3), where the glaciers of the Ice Age originated in the highest part of the Alps and flowed down a very steep gradient into the neighbouring mountains and plains. In the case of the Rhone glacier, huge masses of ice piled up against the chain of the Jura mountains which were directly across its flow. The depth of rock dredged from the Swiss Plateau by glaciation has been estimated at an average of 250 metres over about 1 million years (the Quarternary Period). The Rhone glacier is considered to be the basis of the severe iodine deficiency of the Valais, which is one of the historic areas for the occurrence of goitre and cretinism as described in Chapter 1. It is of interest that the Jura mountains, which were not subject to glaciation, are not deficient in iodine (Merke 1984).

Iodine occurs in the soil and in the sea as iodide. Iodide ions are oxidized by sunlight to elemental iodine, which is volatile, so that every year some 400 000 tons of iodine escape from the surface of the sea. The concentration of iodide in sea water is about 50–60 μg/l. In the air it is approximately 0.7 μg/m^3 The iodine in the atmosphere is returned to the soil by the rain, which has concentrations in the range 1.8–8.5 μg/l. In this way the cycle is completed (Fig. 2.2).

However, the return of the iodine is slow and small in amount compared to the original loss of iodine; and subsequent repeated flooding ensures the continuity of iodine deficiency in the soil. Hence no 'natural correction' can take place, and iodine deficiency persists in the soil indefinitely. All crops grown in these soils will be iodine deficient. As a result, human and animal populations which are totally dependent on food grown in such soil become iodine deficient. The iodine content of plants grown in iodine deficient soils may be as low as 10 μg/kg compared to 1000 μg/kg dry weight in plants in a non-iodine-deficient soil. This accounts for severe iodine deficiency in vast populations in Asia living within systems of subsistence agriculture.

An indication of the iodine content of the soil can be given by the local drinking water concentration. In general, iodine deficient areas have water iodine levels below 2 μg/l as in Nepal and India (0.1–1.2 μg/litre), compared with levels of 9.0 μg/l in the city of Delhi which is not iodine deficient.

The metabolism of iodine in the body

The healthy human adult body contains 15–20 mg of iodine of which 70–80 per cent is in the thyroid gland, which weighs only 15–25 g.

Iodide (chemically bound iodine) is rapidly absorbed through the gut. The normal intake is 100–150 μg per day. Iodine is then excreted by the kidney. The level of excretion correlates well with the level of intake so that it can be used to assess the level of iodine intake. The urinary excretion level, expressed in micrograms per gram of creatinine, is often measured in casual samples to avoid the cumbersome and demanding procedure required for a 24–hour urine collection. Levels of 50 μg/g creatinine or below are indicative of iodine deficiency. A range of values from 20–30 samples provides a good indication of iodine intake and is widely used to monitor the effects of public health programmes (see Chapter 8).

The thyroid has to trap about 60 μg of iodine per day to maintain an adequate supply of thyroxine. This is possible because of the very active iodide trapping mechanism which maintains a gradient of 100:1 between the thyroid cell and the extracellular fluid. In iodine deficiency this gradient may exceed 400:1 in order to maintain the output of thyroxine.

This increased trapping of iodine can be demonstrated using radio-iodine. This was first shown in the Andes by Stanbury and colleagues in 1951. The progressive fall in urinary iodine accompanied by the rise in uptake of I^{131} (radio-iodine) was clearly shown to be an indication of the severity of iodine deficiency. Decreased uptake of I^{131} can be induced by correcting the iodine deficiency with extra 'carrier' iodide with the radio-iodine. Further data demonstrating increased uptake due to iodine deficiency and decreased uptake following injections of iodized oil are shown in Chapter 7 (Table 7.3).

The amount of iodine in the thyroid is closely related to iodine intake. The content may be reduced to only 1 mg or less in the iodine deficient enlarged thyroid (goitre).

Iodine exists in the thyroid as inorganic iodine, in the iodine-containing amino acids: monoiodotyrosine (MIT), diiodotyrosine (DIT), thyroxine (T_4), and triiodothyronine (T_3); in polypeptides containing thyroxine; and in thyroglobulin. Thyroglobulin is a protein which contains the iodized amino acids in a peptide linkage. Thyroglobulin is the chief constituent of the colloid

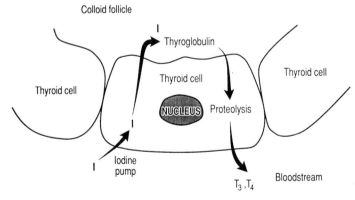

Fig. 2.4. Diagram showing pumping of iodine by the thyroid cell and then passive diffusion into the colloid follicle where it is bound within the protein molecule of thyroglobulin into organic form as the thyroid hormones. The thyroglobulin is then reabsorbed by the cell. It is then broken down to liberate the thyroid hormones which pass into the blood stream.

which fills the thyroid follicle (Fig. 2.4). It is a glycoprotein (contains glucose) with a molecular weight of 650 000. It is the storage form of the thyroid hormones and makes up 90 per cent of the total iodine in the gland.

Iodine exists in the blood as thyroxine (T_4) and triiodothyronine (T_3) and as inorganic iodine. The level of inorganic iodine falls in iodine deficiency and rises with increased intake. T_4 and T_3 are mainly bound to the plasma proteins—only about 0.5 per cent is free in human serum. The level of free T_4 is the important determinant of tissue levels of thyroid hormone. Determination of this free level is therefore the optimum method for assessment of thyroid status and for the diagnosis of reduced thyroid function (hypothyroidism) and increased thyroid function (hyperthyroidism). In the past, determination of total blood organic iodine (mainly thyroxine) was carried out with the plasma protein-bound iodine (PBI) method which gave generally satisfactory results without being as specific as the free T_4 measurement. Other components in the total blood organic iodine which are included in the PBI measurement are T_3 and diiodotyrosine, which comprise less than 10 per cent of the total organic iodine. Increased quantitities of T_3 circulate in iodine deficiency, and an increased amount of the precursor iodotyrosines occurs in the blood in states of hyperthyroidism or following thyroid stimulation.

More recently, the quantities of blood thyroid hormones and TSH, the thyroid stimulating hormone of the pituitary (see next section), have been determined using radioimmunoassay (RIA). Known amounts of radioactively labelled hormones compete with the unknown amount of hormone in the blood in binding to a specific antibody. The technology for these determinations is still advancing.

The advent of automation and computer technology has made it possible to assay large numbers of samples with storage of data and use of quality controls. As we shall see, these advances are of the greatest value for public health programmes when large numbers of samples need to be measured.

Iodine levels in milk are also sensitive to the level of iodine intake. The iodine is present only as iodide. Iodine levels in cow's milk are raised by the recent use of iodophors (iodine-containing antiseptics) in the diary industry. This practice is now widespread in the West.

The production and regulation of the thyroid hormones

The trapping of iodide by the thyroid depends on an active transport mechanism (i.e., requires energy) which is called 'the iodine pump'. This mechanism is regulated by the thyroid stimulating hormone (TSH), thyrotrophin, which is released from the pituitary to regulate thyroid secretion. Other ions can act as competitors—including thiocyanate. Thiocyanate is derived from the metabolism of hydrogen cyanide (HCN) which is found in foods such as cassava, a dietary staple in Zaire and many other countries. This explains the occurrence of goitre and severe hypothyroidism in Zaire (see Chapter 3).

The iodide is released by the thyroid cells into the colloid follicle phase between the cells, where it is oxidized by hydrogen peroxide from the thyroid peroxidase system (Figs. 2.4, 2.5). It then combines with tyrosine in the thyroglobulin to form MIT and DIT. The oxidation process then continues with the coupling of MIT and DIT to form the iodotyrosines (Fig. 2.5). This oxidation process can be readily blocked by various drugs including propylthyrouracil and carbimazole which are widely used for the treatment of hyperthyroidism. There may also be a congenital defect in biosynthesis so that iodide cannot bind to tyrosine—this is a cause of goitre and hypothyroidism which may run in families. Such a defect does not, however, occur in iodine deficient goitre; the reason why iodine deficiency causes goitre in some people and not in others is not known.

Finally, the iodized thyroglobulin, including the iodized amino acids, is absorbed back into the thyroid cells by a process called 'pinocytosis'. It is then exposed to proteolytic enzymes which break it down to release the T_4 and T_3 into the blood (Fig. 2.4). The unused iodotyrosines are conserved for incorporation into a subsequent cycle of the biosynthetic process. With states of thyroid stimulation

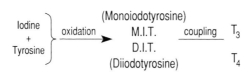

Fig. 2.5. The chemical changes that take place in the formation of thyroxine (T_4) and triiodothyronine (T_3) from iodine and the amino-acid tyrosine within the thyroglobulin molecule.

this conservation process may not be able to keep pace with the production of free iodotyrosines. These may leak into the circulation but have no apparent biological effect.

The regulation of thyroid hormones is a complex process involving not only the thyroid, but the pituitary, the brain, and the peripheral tissues (Fig. 2.6). Thyroid secretion is under the control of the pituitary gland through the thyroid stimulating hormone (TSH). TSH is a glycoprotein with a molecular weight of approximately 28 000. It has two subunits: the 'X subunit' has virtually the same structure as other pituitary hormones, while the β subunit is specific for TSH, but essentially the same across the different animal species.

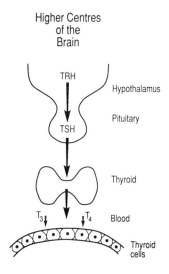

Fig. 2.6. The regulation of the secretion of thyroid hormones by the pituitary through the thyroid stimulating hormone, thyrotrophin (TSH), and the thyrotrophin releasing hormone (TRH).

The action of TSH occurs through the binding of the B subunit to specific receptor sites in the membranes of the thyroid cells. The ensuing sequence of events involves the activation of adenylate cyclase which in turn activates the phosphorylation of various proteins and enzymes within each cell including the nucleus, where one major effect is on gene structures for RNA replication and protein synthesis.

TSH activates all stages of iodine metabolism in the thyroid from trapping to the secretion of T_4 and T_3. Iodide transport is accelerated, there is an increase in the organic binding of iodide in the tyrosine molecules, there is an increase in the coupling rate of MIT and DIT to form T_4 and T_3, and then the pinocytosis of colloid by the thyroid cell leads to the release of T_4 and T_3 into the circulation.

The control of TSH secretion is by a 'feed-back' mechanism related closely to the level of T_4 in the blood (Fig. 2.6). As the blood T_4 falls, the pituitary TSH secretion rises to increase thyroid activity and the output of T_4 into the circulation, and so maintain the necessary level of circulating hormone. If this is not possible, due for example to severe iodine deficiency, then the level of T_4 remains lowered and the level of TSH remains elevated. Both these measurements are used for the diagnosis of hypothyroidism at various stages in life, but particularly in the neonate.

TSH secretion is also under the control of the brain through the thyrotophin releasing hormone (TRH), which is released from the hypothalamus, a small region at the base of the brain (close to the pituitary) which is very important for the control of all the pituitary hormones. TRH is released into the pituitary portal system from where it goes direct to the pituitary. There, it influences the synthesis and release of TSH which is produced by special cells in the anterior lobe of the pituitary (Fig. 2.6). TRH is in turn under the influence of neurotransmitters (adrenalin, noradrenalin, and serotonin, which increase its output, and dopamine, which reduces it). However, TRH is found in high concentrations in various parts of the brain, including the pineal region, and also in the pancreas. This suggests that TRH may have other functions than the control of the thyroid.

Thyroid activity during pregnancy

The thyroid gland is formed from the first part of the gastrointestinal tract (the primitive pharynx) to become a solid organ able to concentrate iodide and secrete the thyroid hormones. Other organs derived from the gastrointestinal tract such as the salivary glands, the breast, the stomach, and the intestinal glands also concentrate iodide but do not secrete thyroid hormones.

In the human, the thyroid has developed by the end of the first 12 weeks of gestation. The pituitary develops over the same period so that TSH becomes available to stimulate the thyroid. The hypothalamus develops from the 10th to 30th weeks. Maturation of neuroendocrine control occurs after the 20th week. Between 18 and 22 weeks TSH can be detected in the blood, followed by a rise in T_4. T_3 remains low due to the preferential formation of reverse T_3 by the 5′deiodinase enzyme, which removes the inner ring 5 iodine atom. Reverse T_3 has no hormonal activity, in contrast to T_3. Just before birth, there is a decline in this enzyme with a rise in 5′deiodinase (outer ring) with a consequent rapid rise in T_3 and fall in reverse T_3 (Fig. 2.1). This change prepares the organism for the transition from intra-uterine life, where there is less demand for oxygen, to extra-uterine life with increased demand for oxygen and the higher rate of metabolism required for survival, for which the thyroid hormones are necessary.

The fetal thyroid is independent of maternal TSH, which is blocked or inactivated by the placenta, as is maternal T_4 and T_3. But there is evidence that maternal T_4 does cross the placental barrier early in pregnancy and is very important to fetal growth and development prior to the function of the fetal thyroid. This question is taken up in detail in Chapter 5.

Fetal development is threatened by the passage of various agents across the placental barrier, including goitrogens, such as thiocyanates, and drugs used in treatment of hyperthyroidism, such as propylthiouracil.

Role of the thyroid in growth and development

Thyroid function is essential to normal growth and development. Thyroid hormone deficiency, whether produced by removal of the thyroid or absence of the thyroid due to disease or congenital defect, is associated with severe retardation of growth and maturation of almost all organ systems. Body weight does not increase and there is retardation of bone growth. These effects can be shown clearly following thyroidectomy in the fetal and neonatal periods, but are also apparent at later stages. The effects are most apparent in tissues that are rapidly proliferating. Measurements of weight and cellular growth by estimation of the DNA content of the tissues reveals retardation in different organs. (See Chapter 5.)

The sensitivity of different organs to thyroid deficiency varies. The brain is particularly susceptible to damage during the fetal and early postnatal period. At birth in the human, the brain is still at a stage of early maturation as indicated by having reached less than a third of its mature weight at that stage. For this reason every new-born child in many Western countries is now checked for the level of thyroid hormones soon after birth (usually by a heel prick sample of blood at the 4th or 5th day) so that if there is any deficiency the level can be made normal by giving replacement therapy with thyroxine. The results of this measure are generally satisfactory, although there is evidence of residual effects even with optimal treatment. IQ decreases sharply when therapy is delayed after the age of three months. However, some patients treated before three months still have a very low IQ. It has now become clear that the result depends on the extent of retardation during fetal life. This can be estimated by determination of bone age. If significant retardation of bone age is evident at birth, the likelihood of completely normal brain development is much less than if the bone age is not retarded.

These effects have been studied extensively in rats following thyroidectomy at different stages. The effect on the brain following thyroidectomy within the first 10 days of life can only be reversed by immediate treatment. But following a thyroidectomy of 40, 70, or 90 days, a delay of 30 days in the start of treatment makes little difference. These results are consistent with clinical observations of human patients with hypothyroidism, which indicate that defects in mental function can usually be completely reversed in adult in contrast to newborn infants, due to the very active growth period of infancy.

The biological effects of thyroid hormones are particularly evident on growth and development. These effects range from the induction of metamorphosis in tadpoles, to the different stages of fetal, neonatal, and child development in animals and man. These effects are probably mediated by action on gene expression with increased synthesis of new proteins and enzymes, or by activation of existing enzymes. An increase in oxygen consumption also occurs in some tissues (liver, kidney, and muscle) but not in others (adult brain).

The mechanism of action of thyroid hormones at the subcellular or molecular level has been the subject of much research and debate in the last 30 years. There are two main schools of thought. The first maintains that the thyroid hormones initiate action at the level of the nucleus. The second maintains that the action is at the plasma membrane and extranuclear structures such as the mitochondria, which are sites of energy production. Conversion of T_4 to T_3 is now generally regarded as essential for the action of the hormones and there is evidence of a high affinity T_3 receptor on cell nuclei. The receptor is a non-histone protein believed to be important in gene expression. There is correlation between T_3 binding to the nucleus and biological responses to thyroid hormones in many tissues. However, this site of action does not exclude other possibilities, including extranuclear sites. High affinity T_3 binding sites have also been described in the mitochondria. Cell membranes (e.g. liver) also have T_3 binding sites. It seems likely that there are a number of sites of action of the thyroid hormones in view of the number and diversity of their effects.

The development of goitre

The preceding discussion on thyroid hormones provides the framework for understanding goitre as a result of iodine deficiency. Although not the only cause, iodine deficiency is the primary cause of goitre. Goitrogens such as thiocyanates can enhance the effect of iodine deficiency; they are referred to as secondary factors.

A remarkable series of experiments were carried out by David Marine over the period 1909–1914 which demonstrated the close relation of iodine to thyroid enlargement and goitre in trout. These studies ranged from mountain trout in Utah, to California (sea trout and sea bass) and pike from Lake Erie. Thyroid enlargement was never found in sea fish but pike from Lake Erie showed varying degrees of hyperplasia. Pike kept in tanks of Lake Erie water also showed thyroid hyperplasia, but reversion to normal took place following the addition of iodide to the water. Subsequent observations on fish farms in various parts of the world have established the necessity of iodine to be in the feed (Marine 1914).

A recent report in the International Zoo Year book (Olney 1988) has described goitre in sharks in Japan. The Oeno Zoological gardens could not keep its sharks alive for very long. Research carried by HRH Prince Mashito (a marine scientist like his illustrious father Hirohito) helped the Zoo to establish that this was the result of efficient filtration removing iodine from the shark's water.

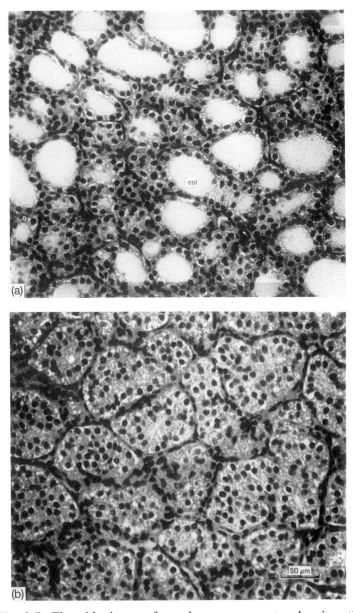

Fig. 2.7. Thyroid tissue of newborn marmosets showing the presence of colloid material in the follicles of the normal control gland (a) compared to its absence in the iodine deficient gland (b) with great increase in size and number of the thyroid cells. (From Mono *et al.* 1986, with permission.)

When goitrous, the sharks stopped feeding and starved to death. Regular iodine addition to the water maintained the sharks in good health!

The basic effect of iodine deficiency is to interfere with the production of thyroid hormones, because iodine is an essential constituent of the T_4 and T_3 molecules. The lowering of output from the thyroid leads to a fall in the blood levels of T_4 but some increase in T_3 preferentially in iodine deficiency).

The fall in the level of T_4 leads to increase in TSH output from the pituitary, increase in uptake of iodide, and increased turnover associated with hyperplasia of the cells of the thyroid follicles. The reserves of colloid containing thyroglobulin are gradually used up so that the gland has a much more cellular appearance than normal (Fig. 2.7). The size of the gland increases with the formation of a goitre. Enlargement is regarded as significant in the human when the size of the lateral lobes is greater than the terminal phalanx of the thumb of the person examined. More precise measurements can now be made using ultrasound.

Chronic severe iodine deficiency is associated with gross thyroid hyperplasia. Goitre increases in prevalence with the severity of the iodine deficiency, and becomes almost universal in a population with an iodine intake less than $10\,\mu g$ per day. Persistent thyroid enlargement leads to the formation of nodules, which are common in longstanding goitres. Various other changes occur including separation (sequestration) of iodine into pools not available for hormone secretion; thus large quantities of abnormal iodine compounds of low molecular weight are resistant to enzymatic digestion. Studies in animals demonstrate impaired iodization of thyroglobulin associated with impaired protein breakdown and a significant escape of non-hormonal iodine, including thyroglobulin, into the blood.

Conclusion

The loss of iodine from the soil due to glaciation, snow, high rainfall, and flooding leads to a low iodine content of all food grown in it. Inadequate dietary iodine leads to reduced synthesis of thyroid hormones, thyroxine (T_4) and triiodothyronine (T_3). The lower level of T_4 in the blood stimulates the pituitary gland to secrete thyrotrophin (TSH). TSH increases the rate of pumping iodine by the thyroid from the blood and the production of the thyroid hormones. There is cell hyperplasia with the enlargement of the thyroid gland that is called a goitre. However, persistence of the deficiency leads to a greater depression of the level of T_4, with the eventual effects of hypothyroidism on growth and mental development.

Bibliography

Marine, D. (1914). *Journal of Experimental Medicine,* **19**, 70.

Merke, F. (1984). *The history and iconography of endemic goitre and cretinism.* MTP Press, Lancaster (originally published by Hans Huber, Berne in 1971).

Olney, P. (ed.) (1988). *International Zoo Yearbook,* Vol. 26, London. (Cited in *New Scientist,* 31 March 1988, p. 54.)

Stanbury, J. B., Brownell, G. L., Riggs, D. S., Perinetti, H., Itoiz, J., and Del Castillo, E. B. (1954). *The adaptation of man to iodine deficiency,* pp. 11–209. Harvard University Press, Cambridge, Mass.

Further reading

For more detailed discussion of the biology and physiology of iodine, the reader is referred to the following:

Dunn, J. T., Pretell, E. A., Daza, C. H., and Viteri, F. E. (eds.) (1986). *Towards the eradication of endemic goiter, cretinism, and iodine deficiency.* Scientific Publication No. 502. PAHO, Washington.

Hetzel, B. S. and Maberly, G. F. (1985). Iodine. In *Trace elements in human and animal nutrition* (ed. Mertz W.), 5th edn, Vol. 2, pp. 139–208. Academic Press, New York.

3

A global review of endemic cretinism

The gradual disappearance of cretinism in Europe in the early decades of the 20th century which was discussed in the first chapter led to the condition being almost forgotten. However, in the 1960s it was 'rediscovered' almost simultaneously in a number of the more remote areas of the world. In the island of New Guinea it was seen in the western part, then under Dutch rule, by a group led by Querido of Leiden in 1961, and in the eastern part which was then under Australian administration, by McCullagh in 1959, and by Hennessy in 1964. In China, Chu found cretins in Chengde, in the hills northeast of Beijing in 1961. Subsequently in Brazil, Lobo and colleagues reported cretinism in 1963 following the original observations by Stanbury and colleagues in Mendoza, Argentina in 1951. In Indonesia Djokomoeljanto reported the condition from Central Java. In India the condition had been lost sight of since the original observations of McCarrison in 1908 and Stott and Gupta in 1934, until Ramalingaswami and colleagues reported it again in 1963. (For detailed references see the review of Pharoah *et al.* 1980.)

The clinical manifestations of the condition in these various parts of the world have now been reported in considerable detail and will be reviewed in this chapter. Field studies of thyroid gland function and iodine metabolism have also been made in many countries. Evidence of the association of cretinism with severe iodine deficiency and high goitre rates has been uniformly reported.

The striking feature of the condition when it was rediscovered was the occurrence of a wide range of defects ranging from individuals with isolated mental deficiency or deaf mutism of varying degree, and a varying severity of paralysis of the arms and legs. But there are also individuals who appear to be normal apart from some coordination defect. This indicates that endemic cretinism is part of a spectrum of defects which can all be seen in the iodine deficient population. Endemic cretinism, we shall see, is a community or population disease and not a disease of individuals.

This would be expected from the environmental cause of iodine deficiency.

The two types of cretinism

The term 'cretinism' has been used over the past century for two different conditions. These are the conditions of cretinism associated with endemic goitre (called 'endemic cretinism') in certain areas of the world, and 'sporadic cretinism', used to refer to congenital hypothyroidism, which is not associated with endemic goitre or iodine deficiency and occurs in all parts of the world. Pharoah *et al.* (1980) review full details of the older historical references which are cited below.

The term 'cretin' was used in England by Curling (1850) and Fagge (1871) to refer to cases of hypothyroidism seen apart from endemic goitre. What struck both these authors was the fact that there was no goitre in these patients, though in other ways, they resembled the goitrous cretins.

Then in England in 1873 W.W. Gull described 'a cretinoid state supervening in adult life', and in 1978 W.M. Ord introduced the name 'myxoedema' for this condition. Subsequently it was recognized by the thyroid surgeons Kocher (1883) and Reverdin (1882) in Switzerland that the effects of total thyroidectomy were similar to those of Ord's 'myxoedema' and to those of endemic cretinism.

The celebrated Professor Sir William Osler in his famous textbook *The principles and practice of medicine* in 1907 stated that 'the changes characteristic of cretinism, endemic as well as sporadic, resulted from the loss of function of the thyroid gland.'

It was McCarrison reporting in 1908 from what was then the north-west frontier of India (now the Karakoram Mountains in Northern Pakistan), who first clearly distinguished two types of endemic cretins—the 'nervous' and the 'myxoedematous'—in a series of 203 patients. In the nervous type he recognized mental defect, deaf mutism, spastic diplegia (paralysis), and a spastic rigidity, usually affecting the legs with a characteristic gait. Squint was also noted. The myxoedematous type had all the characteristics of severe hypothyroidism: dry swollen skin and tongue, deep hoarse voice, apathy, and mental deficiency. This condition McCarrison regarded as identical with 'sporadic cretinism'.

In a later series from Northern India in 1934, Stott and Gupta recorded similar findings in a series of 35 cretins, 50 per cent of whom were deaf mute. They found that the deaf mute subjects were not usually hypothyroid.

The author has been privileged to have the opportunity to study with Chinese colleagues endemic cretinism in the People's Republic of China during three visits in 1981, 1982, and 1984. Approximately one third of the Chinese population live in iodine deficient environments all over China, which is notable for its extensive mountain ranges.

The two types of cretinism are readily seen in China. The neurological type is the predominant form. In Hetian district in Xinjiang, which is only some 300 kilometres East of Gilgit where McCarrison made his original observations in the first decade of the century, I was able to observe a similar situation in 1982, with both neurological, hypothyroid, and mixed types present.

The Hetian district is in the Xinjiang Uighur Autonomous Region of China situated at the foot of the Karakoram Mountains (of Tibet) to the south of the Tarim Basin and the Taklamakan Desert. The

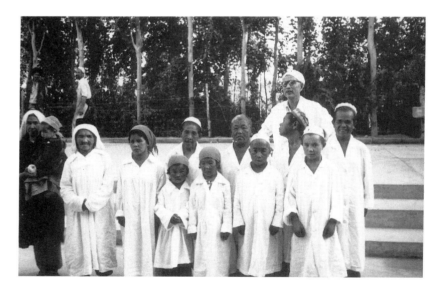

Fig. 3.1. Group of middleaged myxoedematous cretins in Hetian, Sinjiang, China, showing the dwarfism and mask-like faces. Other evidence of gross hypothyroidism included mental torpor, dry skin, and skeletal retardation.

incidence of goitre is 55–57 per cent and that of endemic cretinism 2.1 per cent. In the neighbouring Luofu County, the goitre rate was 46.5 per cent and the cretinism rate 1.8 per cent.

In 1982 a group led by my colleagues Dr Wang Hou-min and Dr Ma Tai presented the results of a study of 72 cretin patients. They spanned an age range of 3–68 years. There were 31 myxoedematous subjects and 21 neurological cases with the other 20 having a mixed clinical presentation (Wang, Ma, Li *et al.* 1983).

The myxoedematous cretins all showed severe hypothyroidism with dwarfism present so that the adult height of 24 adults corresponded to that of normal Uighur children of 9–10 years of age (Fig. 3.1). There was usually gross evidence of skeletal retardation, weak abdominal muscles, inactive bowel function, and delayed tendon reflexes—all classic features of hypothyroidism.

The neurological cretins were not so short in height, with normal muscles and normal bowel function and only one showing some evidence of skeletal retardation (Fig. 3.2).

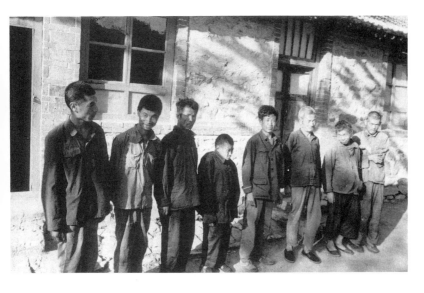

Fig. 3.2. Group of middle-aged neurological cretins from Chengde, China with muscular deformity and mental defects, but no growth retardation (with one exception). There was no clinical evidence of hypothyroidism in these cretins.

In general, mental deficiency was not so severe in the myxoedematous cretins, who showed more self-reliance, and better mental function and calculating ability than was the case with the neurological cretins. Deaf mutism was seen in the neurological cretins but not in the myxoedematous cretins. As would be expected, from their hypothyroidism serum thyroxine levels were lower in the myxoedematous cretins, with elevated TSH in the former. Urine iodine excretion was grossly reduced in all cases. A summary of the differences between the two types is shown in Table 3.1.

Table 3.1 *Comparative clinical features in neurological and hypothyroid cretinism*

Feature	Neurological cretin	Hypothyroid cretin
Mental retardation	Present, often severe	Present, less severe
Deaf-mutism	Usually present	Absent
Cerebral diplegia	Often present	Absent
Stature	Usually normal	Severe growth retardation usual
General features	No physical signs of hypothyroidism	Coarse dry skin, husky voice
Reflexes	Excessively brisk	Delayed relaxation
ECG	Normal	Small voltage QRS complexes and other abnormalities of hypothyroidism
X-ray limbs	Normal	Epiphyseal dysgenesis
Effect of thyroid hormones	No effect	Improvement

Modified from Hetzel and Potter (1983) with permission.

It is apparent that these two types of cretinism are distinct conditions although both are related to iodine deficiency. The features of the myxoedematous type are essentially the same as those of sporadic cretinism, as McCarrison recognized, except for the association with severe iodine deficiency. Sporadic cretinism occurs all over the world whether or not iodine deficiency is present. It is usually found with evidence of an absent or misplaced thyroid or with a congenital defect in the biosynthesis of the hormones. The term 'congenital hypothyroidism' is now generally preferred to sporadic cretinism to prevent confusion. Its incidence is about 3 in 10 000 in Western populations that are receiving adequate iodine.

Cretinism in Europe

Since 1930, studies of cretinism in Europe have been mainly carried out in Switzerland and Italy. The condition has been found primarily in older age groups. In a classic monograph published in 1936, de Quervain and Wegelin described the Swiss cretins in considerable detail and also reviewed the world literature up to that time. They described two groups, one with goitre and one without goitre. The group without goitre showed retarded growth and other features of hypothyroidism. Hearing was usually normal. The thyroid showed atrophy and fibrosis. By contrast, goitrous cretins were of normal height and had neurological features due to cerebral diplegia producing weakness or paralysis of the legs.

Subsequent studies on institutionalized Swiss cretins by König (1968) have revealed mental deficiency with variable degrees of hearing loss but no evidence of dwarfism or hypothyroidism. Severe spastic defects in the legs were sometimes present.

In Northern Italy (Piedmont), extensive laboratory studies have been reported by Costa and his team from Turin in 1964. They studied thyroid function with the help of radioactive iodine and concluded that the endemic cretin was not usually hypothyroid. Myxoedema was seen in only 8 per cent of the patients but nervous features were much more prominent (anomalies of gait, speech, and hearing together with mental deficiency). In a 60-year follow-up of cretins from Northern Italy by Cerletti *et al.* (1963) a series of pictures reveals that a change can occur from a hypothyroid appearance in childhood to a normal thyroid state in the adult. This probably reflects an increase in dietary iodine intake with improvement in thyroid function.

Goitre and cretinism have been reported from Sicily as recently as 1981 in north-eastern Sicily on the north-west side of Mount Etna. Squatrito *et al.* (1981) reported a series of 19 cretins already identified by local doctors in the area as severely mentally retarded. The age range was 15–39 years with one of 60. Nine of them showed clinical and laboratory evidence of hypothyroidism and were therefore myxoedematous cretins. The other ten were clinically euthyroid and had deaf mutism and/or pyramidal tract dysfunction and were neurological cretins. Some familial aggregation was observed. The urinary iodine excretion was very low. These findings indicate the need for control of iodine deficiency.

Cretinism in South America

In 1771 in Argentina, Sanchez Salvador reported: 'In Salta and Jujing you see many people with double chins (called cotes here) which make them stupid and, as they are called here in this country, opas.' In 1805 there were similar reports from the Ecuadorean Andes north of Quito. Subsequent observations from 1950 confirm the predominance of neurological cretins in Ecuador, Argentina, and Venezuela (Pharoah *et al.* 1980). In 1951 Stanbury's group examined 50 cretins in Mendoza. Almost all were mute and in none of them was a clinical diagnosis of hypothyroidism made. In 13 subjects a normal level of serum P B I was demonstrated (Stanbury *et al.* 1954)

Since 1962, more intensive observations in Ecuador by Fierro-Benitez's group confirmed the association of mental retardation and deaf mutism with a higher prevalence of goitre, but general malnutrition associated with gross poverty was also evident (Fierro-Benitez *et al.* 1970). A comparison of 74 cretins (with average IQs of 50) and 104 'normal' persons from the same community revealed a considerable diversity of defects—only 6 of the cretins had normal hearing. A wide spectrum of disorders of gait was apparent: severe muscle spasticity and flexion, internal rotation of the knees, bone deformities such as flattening of the head of the femur, and spinal deformities such as kyphoscoliosis. This had resulted from the spastic muscles. The forehead was usually narrow with saddle nose. Squint was present in 20 per cent.

A similar goitre rate (60 per cent) to that of the total population was found, with similar results for thyroid function tests. Only occasional cretins had definite signs and symptoms of hypothyroidism. When six of the cretins were treated with thyroid hormones over a 5-year period, there was very little improvement apart from slight changes in the skin and hair, with some increase in physical activity. This confirms the irreversible nature of the features of neurological cretinism which was the type seen in about 90 per cent of the cases. Approximately 10 per cent showed a mixture of nervous and hypothyroid features, but no pure myxoedematous cretins were seen as described in Zaire or in China.

Similar observations have been recorded in the states of Goias and Matto Grosso in Brazil (Pharoah *et al.* 1980).

Cretinism in Africa

In Africa, goitre is widespread in association with a hilly and mountainous terrain. Cretinism is in general less severe and extensive than in Asia. However, Zaire has one of the most extensive endemics of cretinism in the world and has been studied by the Belgian group based at the Free University of Brussels (Bastenie *et al.* 1962; Delange *et al.* 1972). Most of the cases are of the myxoedematous variety, in contrast to all other regions of the world. This endemic has been studied in Northern Zaire in the Ubangi region (between the Congo and Zaire rivers, in the Uele, and in the Lake Kivu region, Idjwi Island).

On Idjwi island, 9000 people were examined. The goitre rate was 54 per cent, and 99 cretins were found (1.1 per cent). Only 11 of these were clinically euthyroid and deaf mute, and of these 7 had a

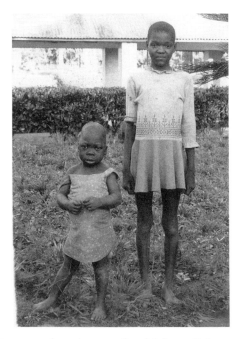

Fig. 3.3. A myxoedematous cretin girl from Zaire aged 9 showing gross dwarfism compared to a normal girl of 9 years. (From Delange *et al.* 1981, with permission.)

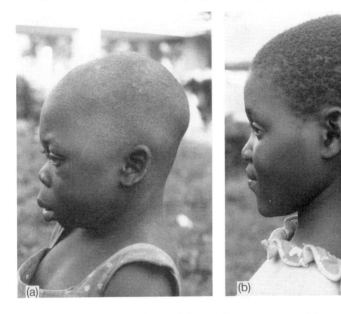

Fig. 3.4a,b. Side view of face of same two subjects as Fig. 3.3 showing the retardation of facial development. (From Delange *et al.* 1981, with permission.)

spastic diplegia. The remaining 88 were myxoedematous cretins with severe hypothyroidism associated with dwarfism, retarded facial development, mental deficiency, dry swollen skin, and umbilical hernia (Fig. 3.3, 3.4).

The diagnosis of severe hypothyroidism was confirmed by biochemical tests—low T_4 and high TSH. X-ray studies (Fig. 3.5) revealed severe skeletal retardation indicative of the onset of hypothyroidism just before birth or in the first few months of life. Severe changes were also observed in the electrocardiagram (low-voltage QRS complexes with flattening of the T-waves) which are typical of hypothyroidism. Similar observations had been made earlier in the Uele district (Bastenie *et al* 1962).

The striking feature of this evidence in Zaire compared to the rest of the world is the overwhelming predominance of severe hypothyroidism. In other parts of Africa cretinism is seen but is much less common and is usually of the neurological type.

The reason for this discrepancy between Zaire and the rest of the

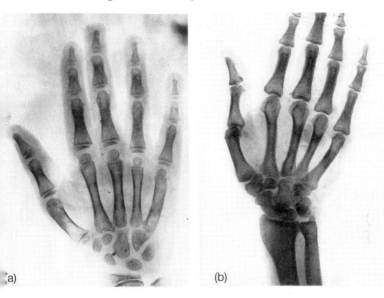

(a)
(b)

Fig. 3.5a,b. X-rays of the wrists of two subjects showing delay in bone formation in a myxoedematous cretin aged 21 compared to the normal subject aged 20. (From Delange *et al.* 1981, with permission.)

world is of great interest and importance. The terrain is fairly flat, covered by equatorial forest, with an altitude of 100 metres above sea level. The climate is hot and humid and the people consume large quantities of cassava as their dietary staple. Evidence is now available that there is an excess quantity of thiocyanate in the blood of these subjects. This results from the detoxification by the liver of cyanide which results from hydrolysis of linamarin from the cassava, in the gut. The thiocyanate causes an excessive loss of iodine through the kidneys. Extensive observations indicate that goitre and myxoedematous cretinism appear when the urine iodide/thiocyanate ratio exceeds 4. In these areas in Zaire it is usually greater than 7. The myxoedematous cretinism probably arises from fetal hypothyroidism produced as a result of cassava consumption by the mother. It is maintained following birth by cyanide ingestion from breast milk. Hence the stage is set for infant hypothyroidism, with severe effects on physical and mental development.

Cretinism in Asia and Oceania

Cretinism is an extensive problem in Asia and Oceania. It is associated with high rates of goitre and severe iodine deficiency in China, India, Indonesia, Nepal, Burma, Pakistan, and Papua New Guinea.

In China the two types have already been described earlier in this chapter. It is of great interest that there appears to be a different geographical localization of the two types. If a line is drawn across China from the north-east to the south-west, only neurological cretins are seen east of this line (as in Guijou, Anhui, and Heilongjiang). Both types occur west of this line (in Sinjiang, Chinghai, and Inner Mongolia). The reasons for this different distribution are quite obscure at this time.

Detailed studies of the myxoedematous cretins in Xinghai province are being made through a China–Australia Collaborative Scientific programme by a group led by Dr Glen Maberly and Dr Creswell Eastman of the Westmead Hospital, Sydney and Dr C. You of the Institute for Endemic Diseases, Qinghai Province. The aim is to try to elucidate the pathological process involved in what appears to be an atrophic state of the thyroid gland described in the earlier literature from Europe. The presence of atrophy has now been confirmed (De Quervain and Wegelin 1936) in older cretins in China using ultrasound studies.

In India in the Himalayan region the predominant type seen is neurological. This is also true of Nepal and Bhutan. In the Terai area in the Ganges valley just to the south of the Himalayas, cretinism is widely prevalent but possibly not quite as severe as in the mountains.

In Indonesia the predominant type seen is also neurological. There are seven hyperendemic areas, including north and west Sumatra, east and central Java, Irian Jaya, Kalimantan, and Bali. In central Java the villages with high rates of goitre are more likely to be on volcanic soil. Preliminary observations indicate a reduced iodine content.

The difference between the cretinism seen in Nepal and that observed in Zaire has been confirmed by the Belgian group, led by Dr F. Delange of Brussels (1981). The high Trisuli and Langtang Valleys of Nepal, approximately 100 kilometres north of Kathmandu, could only be reached by walking. The altitude is 1400–3400

Table 3.2 *Comparison of the epidemiological characteristics of endemic goiter in Northern Zaire (Bambesa District) and in Northern Nepal (Trisuli District).*

Variables	Trisuli District (Nepal)	Bambesa District (Uele–Zaire)
Number of inhabitants surveyed	1658	6416
Fraction of the total population (%)	100	90
Prevalences (%) of		
—All goitres	55.3	64.5
—Visible goitres	28.5	33.0
—Nodular goitres	35.7	30.1
—Endemic cretinism	5.1	2.8
—Myxoedematous	0.5	2.7
—Neurological	4.6	0.1

From Delange *et al.* (1981) with permission.

metres above sea level. A 4-week house-to-house survey of the village of Langtang involved the total population of 1658 inhabitants. In Zaire the area studied was the district of Bambesa in the Uele area. The area is flat, covered by equatorial forest with an altitude only 100 metres above sea level. The climate is hot and humid and the survey covered 6416 people—about 90 per cent of the population of the district. The initial results regarding goitre and cretinism in the two communities are shown in Table 3.2.

Both populations had severe iodine deficiency of similar degree. Casual urine samples for determination of iodine excretion and thiocyanate (SCN) concentration revealed low iodine excretion, with evidence of thiocyanate ingestion in Zaire but not in Nepal.

The criterion for diagnosis of cretinism was mental deficiency as confirmed by the relatives and by the community. The findings confirm that there are two major types of cretinism, hypothyroidism, and the multiple neurological complex.

Out of 84 cretins seen in Nepal, longstanding hypothyroidism was seen in 25. Only 8 of these were found to be normal on neurological examination as was seen in the myxoedematous cretins in Zaire. The other 17 had predominantly neurological signs and symptoms and were considered to be showing the mixed syndrome. Seventy-six of the cretins showed deaf mutism; 38 of these had other neurological effects, while the others showed spastic diplegia (22), increased

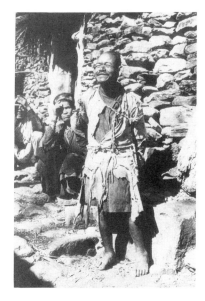

Fig. 3.6. A 47-year-old neurological cretin from Langtang, Nepal, with quadriplegia, mental retardation and deaf mutism. (From Delange *et al.* 1981, with permission.)

reflexes indicating damage to the pyramidal tract (14), and spastic quadriplegia (2) (Fig. 3.6).

Fetal and maternal factors

Deaf mutism, a characteristic feature of neurological cretinism, does not occur in congenital hypothyroidism. On the contrary, extensive reviews have failed to reveal a case of a neurological cretin born to a hypothyroid mother, although congenital anomalies and fetal loss do occur (McMichael *et al.* 1980). Evidence of impaired mental function in childhood has also been described in the children of hypothyroid mothers. On the other hand, congenital hypothyroidism in the fetus can occur without maternal hypothyroidism. More research is required in this area. (DeLong 1987.)

Conclusion

Further research in the precise relationships between iodine deficiency and endemic cretinism is necessary. Our understanding has been assisted by the study of animal models, described in Chapter 5. In the meantime we can conclude that we are dealing with a syndrome of great diversity, ranging from severe hypothyroidism on the one hand to a severe neurological disorder on the other, with many gradations between. Both neurological and hypothyroid cretinism are related to iodine deficiency, but the pathological processes are clearly different.

Bibliography

Bastenie, P.A., Ermans, A.M., Thys, O., Beckers, C., Van Den Schrieck, H.G., and De Visscher, M. (1962). Endemic goiter in Uele region. III. Endemic cretinism. *Journal of Clinical Endocrinology,* **22**, 187–94.

Cerletti, U., Costa, A., Marocco, F., Masini, A., and Mortara, M. (1963). L'endemia di gozzo-cretinismo oggi e sessanta anni fa. Rilievi nella Valtellina, nella Valle del Mera e nella Val Bisagno. *Ric. Sci.* **33**, (II-A) 5–35.

Costa, A., Cottino, F., Mortara, M., and Vogliazzo (1964). Endemic cretinism in Piedmont. *Panminerva Med.* **6**, 250–9.

Delange, F., Ermans, A.M., Vis, H.L., and Stanbury, J.B. (1972). Endemic cretinism in Idjwi Island. (Kivu Lake, Republic of Congo). *Journal of Clinical Endocrinology and Metabolism* **34**, 1059–66.

——, Valeix, P., Bourdoux, P., Lagasse, R., Ermans, J.P., Thilly, C., and Ermans, A.M. (1981). Comparison of the epidemiological and clinical aspects of endemic cretinism in Central Africa and in the Himalayas. In *Recent approaches to the problems of mental deficiency* (eds. B.S. Hetzel and R.M. Smith), pp. 243–64. Elsevier, Amsterdam.

DeLong, R. (1987). Neurological involvement in iodine deficiency disorders. In *The prevention and control of iodine deficiency disorders* (eds. B.S. Hetzel, J.B. Stanbury, and J.T. Dunn) pp. 49–63, Elsevier, Amsterdam.

De Quervain, F. and Wegelin, C. (1936). Der endemische kretinismus. Springer, Berlin.

Fierro-Benitez, R., Stanbury, J.B., Querido, A., De Groot, L., Alban, R., and Endova, J. (1970). Endemic cretinism in the Andean region of Ecuador. *Journal of Clinical Endocrinology and Metabolism* **30**, 228–36.

Hetzel, B.S. and Pharoah, P.O.D. (eds.) (1971). *Endemic cretinism.* Institute of Human Biology, Goroka, Papua New Guinea.

Hetzel, B.S. and Potter, B.J. (1983). Iodine deficiency and the role of thyroid hormones in brain development. In *Neurobiology of the trace elements* (eds. I. Dreosti and R.M. Smith), pp. 83–133. Humana Press, New Jersey.

König, M.P. (1968). Die kongenitale Hypothyreose und der endemische Kretinismus. Springer, Berlin.

McCarrison, R. (1908). Observations on endemic cretinism in the Chitral and Gilgit Valleys. *Lancet* **2**: 1275–80.

McMichael, A.J., Potter, J.D., and Hetzel, B.S. (1980). Iodine deficiency, thyroid function and reproductive failure. In *Endemic goiter and endemic cretinism* (eds. J.B. Stanbury and B.S. Hetzel), pp. 445–60. Wiley, New York.

Pharoah, P.O.D., Delange, F., Fierro-Benitez, R., and Stanbury, J.B. (1980). Endemic cretinism. In *Endemic goiter and endemic cretinism* (eds. J.B. Stanbury and B.S. Hetzel), pp. 395–421. Wiley, New York.

Squatrito, S., Delange, F., Trimarchi, F., Lisi, E., and Vigneri, R. (1981). Endemic cretinism in Sicily. *J. Endocrinol. Invest.* **4**, 295–302.

Stanbury, J.B., Brownell, G.L., Riggs, D.S., Perinetti, H., Itoiz, J., and Del Castillo, E.B. (1954). *The adaptation of man to iodine deficiency.* Harvard University Press, Cambridge, Mass.

Stott, H. and Gupta, J.P. (1934). The distribution of goitre in the United Provinces. *Indian Journal of Medical Research* **31**, 655.

Wang Hou-min, Ma Tai, Li Xi-tian, Jiang Xin-min, Wang Yan-you, Chen Bin-zhong, Wang Feng-rei, Gao Shi-mei, Ma Ling-yuen, and Su Mayo-yi (1983). A comparative study of endemic myxedematous and neurological cretinism in Hetian and Luopu, China. In *Current problems in thyroid research* (eds. N. Ui, K. Torizuka, S. Nagataki, and K. Miyai), pp. 349–55. Excerpta Medica, Amsterdam.

Further reading

Dunn, J.T., Pretell, E.A., Daza, C.H., and Viteri F.E. (eds.) (1986). *Towards the eradication of endemic goiter, cretinism, and iodine defi-*

ciency. Scientific Publication No. 502. P A H O, Washington.

Hetzel, B.S. and Smith, R.M. (eds.) (1981). *Fetal brain disorders: recent approaches to the problem of mental deficiency*. Elsevier, Amsterdam.

Stanbury, J.B. and Hetzel, B.S. (eds.) (1980). *Endemic goiter and endemic cretinism: iodine nutrition in health and disease*. Wiley, New York.

—— and Kroc, R.L. (eds.) (1972). *Human development and the thyroid gland*. Plenum Press, New York.

4

The evidence from Papua New Guinea

New Guinea is a large, highly mountainous island situated to the north of Australia and at the eastern end of the Indonesian Archipelago. The people are split into many tribal groups with 360 different dialects. The tribal groups are largely incomprehensible to one another, as they live in villages cut off physically from one another.

The people live by the 'slash and burn' economy, clearing the forest by burning the trees, and then cultivating their crops of yams, taro, and in the last 350 years, the sweet potato. The villagers do rely entirely on food grown in these areas around the village (Fig. 4.1). The growing of the sweet potato was associated with a big increase in population and migration to higher altitudes, up to 1000 metres.

The supply of protein by the sweet potato is greater than that from the other vegetables. However, nutrition is not adequate for the level of growth and development seen in the West. Stature is

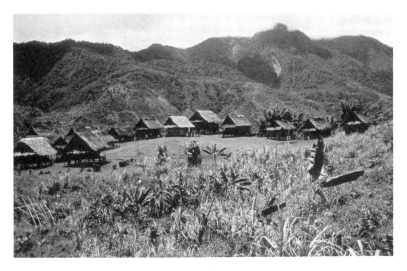

Fig. 4.1. A typical highland village, Gumbot, in the Huon Peninsula Area, Morobe Subdistrict, Papua New Guinea.

stunted, puberty is delayed to approximately 20 years, and there is a loss of muscle mass in middle-age. All of these variations can be attributed to protein deficiency. The addition of protein supplements has been shown to improve growth and reduce the age of puberty. There is a very low intake of salt, but a high intake of potassium. Meat is only rarely available at special feasts once every two years or more in some areas, and not at all in others. This vegetarian diet is associated with a very low intake of fat, a high intake of fibre, and only just enough energy for the vigorous way of life imposed by the environment conditions. Cause of death is most frequently pneumonia, malaria, infection, or injury.

The New Guinea villager living in the mountains is free of vascular disease, has low blood pressure, and is not diabetic. However, his health undergoes a dramatic change when he or she moves to the towns, especially if a salary is available. This permits adoption of a Western style diet high in fat, sugar, and alcohol, which rapidly leads to obesity in association with the more sedentary lifestyle. Blood pressure rises and coronary heart disease starts to appear. Apparently the Melanesian is genetically resistant to the diabetes

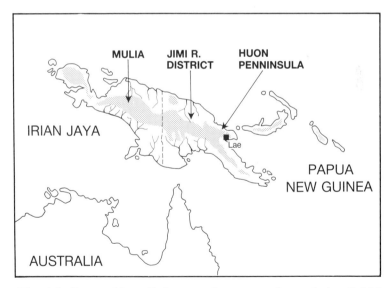

Fig. 4.2. Papua New Guinea, today a member of the British Commonwealth of Nations. The major areas of iodine deficiency and goitre are shaded.

mellitus which occurs so readily under the same conditions in many other Pacific peoples (e.g. Nauru) and in the Australian aborigine.

In the late 19th century, New Guinea was divided by the colonial powers. The western half, known as West New Guinea or West Irian, and now the province of Indonesia, called Irian Jaya, was under Dutch administration until 1961. The eastern half was divided between Germany and Britain until after the First World War when the League of Nations took over the northern part, the southern part remaining as the British Territory of Papua administered by Australia. After the Second World War, Australia took over administration of the northern part from the United Nations in addition to the continuing administration of Papua. Independence of the Territories was achieved in 1976 when Papua New Guinea became a member of the British Commonwealth of Nations (Fig. 4.2). Australia continues to supply substantial aid to Papua

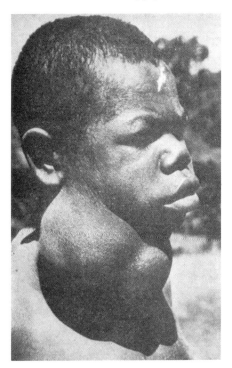

Fig. 4.3. Young New Guinean woman with a large goitre. (From Hetzel 1970, with permission.)

New Guinea: at present (for 1985–6) $320 million per year, approximately one third of its total aid budget.

Between 1945 and 1976, Australia was essentially governing Papua New Guinea. This included responsibility for law and order, health, and education, and economic development. A University was established in Port Moresby in 1966, and an Institute of Technology (now a University of Technology) in Lae in 1967.

The island experiences a high rainfall—up to 240 inches in the Saruwaged mountains north of Lae in the Huon Peninsula. This leads to fast flowing rivers which take topsoil and iodine down to the sea. The mountains are steep, ranging in height up to 4000 metres. Human habitation does not occur above about 1000 metres. However, up to this altitude many live in picturesque villages of thatched houses, with their surrounding vegetable plots in which the soil may be assumed to be iodine deficient (Fig. 4.1).

In this environment there is a high rate of goitre and cretinism (Fig. 4.3). There is evidence of intense hyperplasia of the thyroid (Fig. 4.4). The goitre rate increases with altitude (Fig. 4.5). Cretinism occurs, as it does elsewhere, when the goitre rate increases

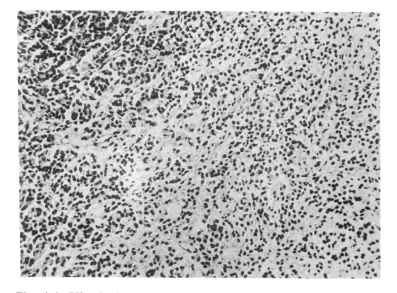

Fig. 4.4. Histological section of large goitre removed because of pressure symptoms, showing intense hyperplasia with no colloid. (From Buttfield and Hetzel 1967, with permission.)

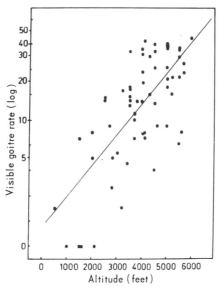

Fig. 4.5. Relation between visible goitre rate in individual villages and altitude. (From Buttfield and Hetzel 1967, with permission.)

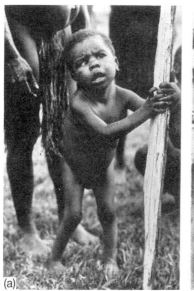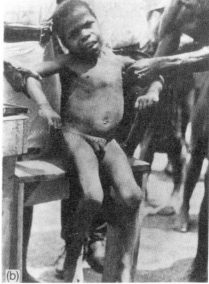

(a)   (b)

above 30 per cent. Cretins may account for 1–10 per cent of the population of individual villages.

The clinical picture of cretinism as first observed by McCullagh (1963*b*) and Hennessy (1964) was essentially that of neurological cretinism with mental deficiency, deaf mutism, spastic paralysis, and squint (Fig. 4.6a,b).

Table 4.1 shows the clinical features observed by Buttfield and Hetzel in a series of 254 cretins living in the Boana area of the Huon Peninsula. Deafness was the most common feature. Definite hypothyroidism was not seen. These cretins, called 'long longs' in Pidgin English, are cared for by people with shelters. They perform simple tasks but soon become incapacitated and die early from pneumonia or other infections.

Similar features of people living in the Mulia area of West New Guinea (now Irian Jaya) were reported by the Dutch group led by Querido (Choufoer *et al.* 1965). It was apparent to the Dutch group as to McCullagh that there was a spectrum of abnormalities. The

Table 4.1 *Endemic cretinism in Papua New Guinea*

Clinical features	
Males	129 (51%)
Females	125 (49%)
Total	254
Visible goitre rate	66 (26%)
Deaf mutism (partial and complete)	177 (70%)
Characteristic vacant faces	161 (64%)
Brisk reflexes	156 (61%)
Extensor plantar response	122 (48%)
Mental abnormalities	120 (47%)
Flexural deformities	70 (28%)
Muscular incoordination	65 (26%)
Dwarfism	65 (26%)

From Buttfield and Hetzel (1969), with permission.

←**Fig. 4.6** (a) A young cretin with squint, ataxia and mental deficiency. (b) A boy of approximately ten years in an area of less severe endemic cretinism suffering from incoordination, ataxia, and mental deficiency. (From Hetzel and Pharoah 1971, with permission.)

condition was a 'community disease' and not due to individual idiosyncrasy.

The occurrence of these abnormalities was something of a shock to these earlier observers. The condition had been essentially 'forgotten' since the early descriptions of McCarrison, from what was then known as the Northwest Frontier of India, published in the *Lancet* in 1908. When they consulted the scientific literature in the early 1960s there was only McCarrison's report to guide them. (The same applied to the Chinese group led by the late Professor H I Chu when they observed cretins in Chengde, North East of Beijing in 1962.) The two clinical pictures of neurological and myxoedematous or hypothyroid cretinism originally reported by McCarrison in 1908 were confirmed. But it was clear that neurological cretinism was by far the most common form of the condition and that the hypothyroid form predominated only in Zaire.

As already pointed out in Chapter 1, there was controversy about the relation of iodine deficiency to neurological cretinism. Its apparent 'spontaneous' disappearance in Southern Europe without any iodized salt program suggested that it was unrelated to iodine deficiency. In 1964 it became apparent that there was an opportunity to investigate this question in New Guinea. This depended on the availability of a new method for the correction of iodine deficiency, namely injections of iodized oil (lipiodol). We now turn our attention to this development, as it has been very important to the whole subject of the prevention and control of the effects of iodine deficiency.

The development of the iodized oil injection

The suggestion that iodized oil might be useful for the control of goitre in Papua New Guinea was made by a chest specialist, Dr Douglas Jamieson, in the late 1950s. He was familiar with the use of iodized oil as a radio-opaque dye to help show cavities in X-rays of the lungs most often due to tuberculosis, a condition that appeared in the New Guinea population following the coming of the white man. After the injection into the body, the dye was well-known to persist for a number of years and to interfere with tests for iodine-containing thyroid hormones in the blood.

Jamieson suggested to Dr John Gunther, then Director of Public Health in Papua New Guinea, that the injection of lipiodol could

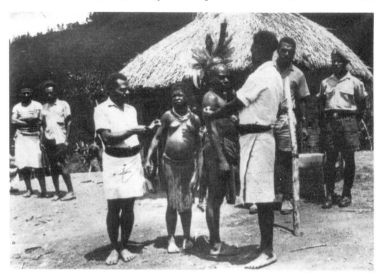

Fig. 4.7. Injection of iodized oil in a Highland village in New Guinea. (From Hetzel and Pharoah 1971, with permission.)

be helpful in the prevention and treatment of goitre. Gunther decided that it was worth a trial and he asked one of the young medical officers in the Public Health Department, Dr Terry McCullagh, to carry out a clinical trial (Fig. 4.7).

First of all, a study was done in Melbourne to see what the effect of the oil was on the thyroid gland. A dose of 4 ml (providing 2 g of iodine) was given to a few volunteers. Measurements were made on the serum protein bound iodine (PBI), the best technique available at that time for measurement of the blood thyroid hormone level, and on the uptake of radioactive iodine (I^{131}) by the thyroid gland. The results indicated persistent effects over 2 years, and it was decided to proceed with further observations in New Guinea. (Clarke *et al.* 1960)

The Boana area in the Huon Peninsula (north of Lae) (Fig. 4.2) was selected for the initial trial. This was a mountainous area with a high rate of goitre in many villages, readily accessible (some 15 minutes) by air from Lae through the airstrip at Boana. In addition there was a well-established Lutheran mission in Boana under the supervision of Reverend and Mrs F. Bergmann from Nuremberg.

The Bergmanns had helped the people to establish the production of coffee beans. They had an excellent working relationship with them, and their help throughout the iodized oil studies was of the greatest value.

McCullagh carried out a controlled trial of the iodized oil by making a comparison with an injection of a salt solution. (McCullagh 1963*a*) Alternate subjects from a number of the villages were injected with iodized oil or the salt solution. Those with obvious goitre were excluded. The people cooperated well with the injections because they had already experienced the benefits of injections (neoarsphenamine) for the cure of Yaws, an unpleasant condition causing unsightly lumps on the legs due to a spirochaetal infection. One injection was sufficient to produce a dramatic cure of Yaws.

After a three-year period, McCullagh carried out a goitre survey of the villages without knowing who had received the oil or the salt injections. He then tabulated the results which revealed an unmistakable effect—the injection of iodized oil had indeed protected against the development of goitre.

McCullagh submitted his findings in a series of papers to the *Medical Journal of Australia* in 1963. I was asked to review the papers and was immediately impressed with the importance of the results. McCullagh remarked at the conclusion of his discussion: 'In spite of the observed effect of iodized oil, there was no more reason to connect iodine deficiency with goitre than quinine deficiency with malaria.' This remark challenged me to investigate two major questions:

(1) Was goitre in New Guinea due to iodine deficiency? and
(2) If so, how effective was the iodized oil in its correction?

Both these questions could only be settled by laboratory investigation involving determinations of thyroid function, and iodine measurements in the urine. In late 1963, I made a research proposal to the New Guinea Medical Research Advisory Committee which was accepted.

With the support of the Head of the Department of Medicine at the University of Adelaide, the late Professor (subsequently Sir Hugh) Robson, I was able to secure a junior research fellowship to which I appointed Dr Ian Buttfield, a recent Adelaide graduate, who together with my laboratory staff, Dr Brian Good, Miss Margaret

Isaachsen, Dr Maurice Wellby, and Miss Enid Mason, made up an excellent team.

After a period of training, Buttfield proceeded to New Guinea in 1964 where he established a good working relationship with Reverend and Mrs Bergmann. It had been decided to follow up the same population as that investigated by McCullagh. It would provide both untreated subjects and subjects who had received the iodized oil injections. Buttfield made rapid progress. In addition to collecting samples of blood and urine for the Adelaide laboratory, he carried out determinations of radio-iodine uptake in the field using transistorized equipment that could be carried in patrol boxes through the mountains.

By early 1965 a substantial amount of data could be analysed. This revealed that there was severe iodine deficiency as indicated by very low levels of urine iodine excretion and low levels of thyroid

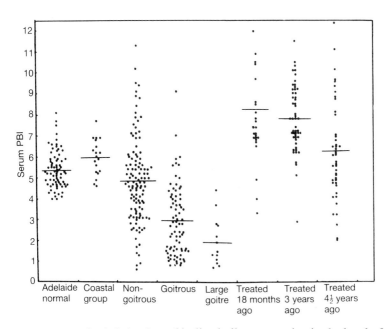

Fig. 4.8. A single injection of iodized oil causes a rise in the level of serum thyroid hormone, as measured by protein-bound iodine (PBI), for $4\frac{1}{2}$ years. Each dot represents an individual. The lines show the mean level for each group. (From Buttfield and Hetzel 1967, with permission.)

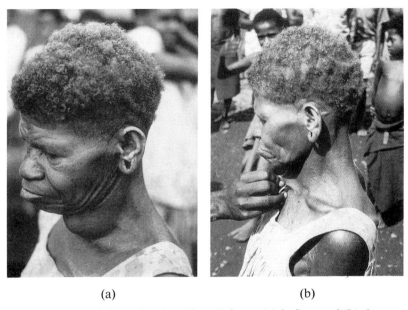

(a)   (b)

Fig. 4.9. Nodular goitre in a New Guinean (a) before and (b) three months after injection of iodized oil. (From Buttfield and Hetzel 1967, with permission.)

hormones in blood—lower in those with goitre, lowest in those with the biggest goitres (Fig. 4.8). Injection of iodized oil had raised the thyroid hormone levels for as long as 3 years after the injection. Subsequently this was shown to extend to 4½ years (Fig. 4.8). One of the striking benefits was the subsidence of goitre subsequent to the injection of iodized oil (Fig. 4.9). This was obviously appreciated by the people, who soon presented themselves at health centres and hospitals requesting the injections. Previously, some of the large goitres which had produced severe pressure symptoms in the neck had been removed surgically. This was a difficult operation because of the greatly increased amount of blood in the gland. After iodized oil injections became established, surgery was no longer required for goitre in New Guinea.

I reported these findings to the 5th International Thyroid Congress in Rome in July 1965. There was considerable interest by those working in the other goitrous areas of the world, particularly Zaire, India, and South America. This led to similar investigations with oil in Zaire, Ecuador, and Peru. The oil had also been used by the Dutch group in West New Guinea, but they were unable to follow the effects until much later due to the Indonesian Revolution.

The New Guinea work was presented to a meeting at Puebla, Mexico in 1969. Through these meetings, iodized oil became well known and used in various countries. We published a comprehensive account of our findings in the *Bulletin of the World Health Organization*, in 1967. Following this, the iodized oil injection was incorporated into the international public health practice of the WHO and UNICEFF.

The prevention of endemic cretinism by injections of iodized oil

We can now return to the subject of endemic cretinism. In 1964 we gained the impression that those villages which had previously had injections of iodized oil no longer had so many cretins. This was clearly very important but required another controlled trial to be certain. If it were so, then the relation of iodine deficiency to cretinism would be established. I put a further proposal to the New Guinea Medical Research Advisory Committee and to the Director of the Public Health Department, Dr Roy Scragg, who agreed to cooperate in the trial. As he pointed out, it was not possible to inject every iodine deficient individual in New Guinea at once. It was not inappropriate therefore to withhold the injection from a group to enable a scientifically controlled trial to be carried out. This position would be more strongly challenged today than it was in 1966.

For this trial, the Jimi River District north of Mount Hagen in the Western Highlands was chosen. It was an area where cretinism was prevalent, particularly in younger age groups, access was available by air and the missions (both Anglican and Lutheran in this case) were cooperative. Dr Peter Pharoah, an experienced New Guinea medical officer, carried out the follow-up at my special request to Dr. Spragg.

The task facing us was much more difficult than in the case of prevention of goitre. It was necessary to establish criteria for the diagnosis of cretinism in young infants. This had not been done before. For this purpose, Pharoah, with great skill, developed a clinical assessment based on motor milestones (sitting, standing, walking), deafness, and squint. These proved satisfactory for a survey of a large population of children.

The trial was set up at the time of the first census in New Guinea in September 1966. Alternate families were given injections of iodized oil or saline. Follow-up was then carried out by Pharoah by regular patrols over the succeeding 5 years. This involved extensive mountain climbing to reach remote villages. It was impossible to cover the whole population of 8000 originally injected. Instead he concentrated on a series of 8 villages where good records could be kept. Pharoah made an assessment of all children born to mothers without knowing who had received iodized oil or saline. This was most important, as the clinical diagnosis was not precise and bias could readily have occurred. Subsequent follow-up has confirmed diagnoses of cretinism in these cases.

Table 4.2   *Pregnancy outcome in the controlled trial of iodized oil in the Western Highlands of Papua New Guinea (Jimi River District)*

	Births	*Children examined*	*Normals*	*Deaths*	*Cretins**
Untreated	534	406	380	97[++]	26[+++]
Iodized oil	498	412	405	66[++]	7[+++]

* Pregnancies were already established when mothers were injected with iodized oil (6 cases) or with saline (5 cases).
[++] P < 0.05
[+++] P < 0.001

From Pharoah *et al.* (1971), with permission.

The initial results of the follow-up became available by the end of 1969 and are shown in Table 4.2 and Fig. 4.10. They indicate that cretins had disappeared from the offspring of mothers who had received iodized oil injections, but continued to appear in those who had received saline. Six cretins had appeared following iodized oil injection but in all except one case, the mother had been noted to be pregnant at the time of the injection. In the other case, there was some doubt about the precise date of birth and she may well have also been pregnant when injected. It was concluded that the injection of iodized oil before pregnancy would prevent cretinism.

These findings were reported to the 6th International Thyroid Congress in Vienna in 1970. They created immediate interest, and when published in the *Lancet* early in 1971, were accepted as defini-

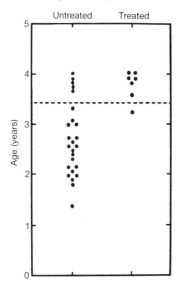

Fig. 4.10. The results of a controlled trial of iodized oil injection in the Jimi River District of the Highlands of Papua New Guinea. Alternate mothers were given an injection of iodized oil and saline in September 1966. All newborn children were followed up for the next five years. Each dot represents a cretin child. The figure shows that mothers given iodized oil injections do not have subsequent cretin children, in comparison with their persistence in the untreated group. (From Pharoah *et al.* 1971, with permission.)

tive at a symposium held at the Institute of Human Biology, Goroka, New Guinea (Hetzel and Pharoah 1971). A subsequent Editorial (*Lancet* 1972) pointed out that the long-standing controversy was now resolved. It could be assumed that the apparent diappearance of cretinism in Southern Europe could be attributed to an increase in dietary intake of iodine as a result of economic development leading to diversification of the food supply.

The findings have been confirmed in other parts of the world although no further controlled trails have been carried out. They would not be feasible and can no longer be ethically justified for this purpose.

Other effects that can be prevented by iodized oil

Another result of the controlled trial was reduction in infant deaths in the treated group (Table 4.2). This indicates an effect of iodine deficiency on survival of the fetus. It expands the concept of iodine deficiency beyond that of goitre and cretinism to that of stillbirths and infant mortality. We shall return to this aspect in later chapters. However, a subsequent follow up study by Pharoah *et al.* (1976) has demonstrated the importance of the level of maternal thyroid hormone (T_4) to both the survival of the pregnancy and cretinism. The lowest range of T_4 (< 25 mg/ml) was associated with a much higher rate of infant deaths and cretinism than levels of maternal $T_4 > 25$ mg/ml.

Further follow-up studies on the same group were carried out by Pharoah after 1976 in collaboration with Professor Kevin Connolly, of the Psychology Department at the University of Sheffield, and myself (Connolly *et al.* 1979). The question arose as to whether there was a continuum of effects of iodine deficiency on brain development that could be prevented by the injection of iodized oil, or simply the one effect of cretinism.

The problem could be approached using measures of intelligence, but appropriate tests were not readily available for New Guinea children who came from a unique cultural background. With the help of Mr Malcolm Hutton, of the Department of Psychological Services in New Guinea, the Pacific Performance Scale of Ord was used. This had been used previously in New Guinea to select police recruits from candidates with no more than a primary school education. Connolly also devised simple measures of psychomotor performance, such as threading beads and using a pegboard, which were found to be discriminatory in preliminary trials with the New Guinea children. (The alternative task of tightening a nut was found to be quite incomprehensible to New Guinea children and hence quite useless for testing purposes.)

A group of children were then tested by Connolly in the Jimi River district without knowledge as to whether they had been exposed to iodine deficiency in pregnancy. It was found that those children exposed to iodine deficiency, aged by this time 10–12 years, did not perform as well in the psychomotor tests as those not exposed to iodine deficiency in pregnancy as a result of their mothers receiving an injection of iodized oil. The differences in performance on the Ord Pacific Performance Test were not as striking. It was of interest to see whether the level of maternal thyroid hormone during pregnancy was significant in relation to these psychomotor test results. Indeed it was later shown that the performance was related significantly to the level of maternal T_4 (Pharoah *et al.* 1984).

The above results therefore indicate the importance of maternal thyroid hormones to fetal brain development. These findings have led to the experimental studies to be described in the next chapter. Taken with the previous trial, these studies reveal a broad spectrum of effects on fetal development, ranging from mortality to cretinism, and psychomotor defects in apparently normal children. This means that a much higher proportion of the iodine deficient population is affected than had previously been thought. We shall be returning to this question again in Chapter 6.

The control of severe iodine deficiency in Papua New Guinea

The investigations described in this chapter indicated the urgent need for correction of iodine deficiency. This was achieved with an iodized oil injection campaign in 1971 and 1972 shortly after completion of the controlled trial in the Western Highlands. Some 120 000 people living in the Highland villages were injected by the Aide Post Orderly (APO), the basic village health worker of the Papua New Guinea Public Health Department.

The APO was trained in a short course over a year to provide simple preventive and curative care for about seven villages comprising a population of some 1000 people. He made a regular circuit on foot and was the key figure in the major reduction in infant mortality achieved over the period from 1952 to 1970. These measures were followed up in 1974 by the passage of legislation making compulsory the iodization of all salt for human consumption.

From 1974 to 1980 Papua New Guinea went through a period of unprecendented prosperity due to high copper and coffee prices. This led to the import of a wide variety of canned foods, including tinned fish from Japan, an excellent source of iodine. It was widely reported that goitre had disappeared from Papua New Guinea. However, following a serious economic recession associated with a steep fall in copper prices, goitre has reappeared in the more remote valleys.

New studies are being carried out by Dr Peter Heywood of the Papua New Guinea Institute of Medical Research in collaboration with Dr Buttfield and myself. Observations on urine iodine levels indicate that moderate iodine deficiency has recurred. This should be controlled as soon as possible to avoid the development of severe iodine deficiency.

To conclude, the story of Papua New Guinea is unique in that the iodized oil injection was introduced and shown to be effective. The value of this measure has been confirmed in Asia (6 million injections in Indonesia, 2 million in Burma, 2 million in Nepal, 2–3 million in China) and in Africa (1½ million injections in Zaire).

The controlled trial has also confirmed the broader spectrum of effects of severe iodine deficiency that had been suspected previously. All these effects can be prevented. (See Chapter 5.)

Finally, a successful public health program was introduced, but the more recent observations indicate some loss of control associated with economic recession. We shall see that this has happened elsewhere in the world. It indicates the need for continued monitoring and surveillance for the effects of iodine deficiency in the populations at risk.

Bibliography

Buttfield, I. H. and Hetzel, B. S. (1967). Endemic goitre in Eastern New Guinea with special reference to the use of iodised oil in prophylaxis and treatment. *Bulletin World Health Organization* **36**, 243–62.

Buttfield, I. H. and Hetzel, B. S. (1969). Endemic cretinism in Eastern New Guinea. *Australasian Annals of Medicine* **18**, 217–21.

Choufoer, J. C., van Rhijn, M., and Querido, A. (1965). Endemic goitre in Western New Guinea. II. Clinical picture, incidence and pathogenesis of endemic cretinism. *Journal of Clinical Endocrinology* **25** 385–402.

Clarke, K. H., McCullagh, S. F., and Winikoff, D. (1960). The use of an intramuscular depot of iodized oil as a long-lasting source of iodine. *Medical Journal of Australia* **1**, 89–91.

Connolly, K. J., Pharoah, P. O. D., and Hetzel, B. S. (1979). Fetal iodine deficiency and motor performance during childhood. *Lancet* **2** 1149–51.

Hennessy, W. B. (1964). Goitre: prophylaxis in New Guinea with intramuscular injections of iodized oil. *Medical Journal of Australia* **1**, 505.

Hetzel, B. S. (1970). The control of iodine deficiency. *Medical Journal of Australia* **2**, 615–22.

Hetzel, B. S. and Pharoah, P. O. D. (eds.) (1971). *Endemic cretinism*. Institute of Human Biology, Papua New Guinea. Monograph Series No. 2.

Lancet editorial (1972). New light on endemic cretinism. *Lancet* **2**, 365–6.

McCarrison, R. (1908). Observations on endemic cretinism in the Chitral and Gilgit valleys. *Lancet* **2**, 1275–80.

McCullagh, S. F. (1963*a*). The Huon Peninsula endemic: I the effectiveness of an intramuscular depot of iodized oil in the control of endemic goitre. *Medical Journal of Australia* **1**, 767–9.

McCullagh, S. F. (1963*b*). The Huon Peninsula endemic: IV endemic goitre and congenital defect. *Medical Journal of Australia* **1**, 884–90.

Pharoah, P. O. D. and Connolly, K. C. (1987). A controlled trial of iodinated oil for the prevention of endemic cretinism: a long term follow-up. *International Journal of Epidemiology* **16**, 68–73.

Pharoah, P. O. D., Buttfield, I. H., and Hetzel, B. S. (1971). Neurological damage to the fetus resulting from severe iodine deficiency during pregnancy. *Lancet* **1**, 308–10.

Pharoah, P. O. D., Ellis, S. M., Ekins, R. P. and Williams, E. S. (1976). Maternal thyroid function, iodine deficiency and fetal development. *Clinical Endocrinology* **5**, 159–66.

Pharoah, P. O. D., Connolly, K. J., Ekins, R. P. and Harding, A. G. (1984). Maternal thyroid hormone levels in pregnancy and the subsequent cognitive and motor performance of the children. *Clinical Endocrinology* **21**, 265–70.

Further reading

Hetzel, B. S. and Pharoah, P. O. D. (eds.) (1971). *Endemic cretinism*. Institute of Human Biology, Papua New Guinea.

Stanbury, J. B. and Hetzel, B. S. (eds.) (1980). *Endemic goitre and endemic cretinism: iodine nutrition in health and disease*. Wiley, New York.

5

The evidence from animal studies

The studies of iodine deficiency in animals complement the studies in human subjects. Animal studies have been of special importance to the earlier study of goitre, and more recently to the study of the effects on the brain. These studies allow observations to be made on individual organs which could not be carried out in humans.

Many observations on naturally occurring iodine deficiency have been made on farm animals in which reproductive failure due to thyroid insufficiency has been recognized for many years. In areas of iodine deficiency, neonates are frequently stillborn, weak, or hairless. Retarded or arrested development of the fetus has occurred at some stage in gestation, resulting in early death and resorption, abortion, stillbirth, or the birth of weak offspring associated with prolonged gestation and parturition and with retention of placental membranes. Subnormal thyroid hormone levels in herds of cattle have been associated with a high incidence of aborted, stillborn, or weak calves. Thyroidectomy of ewes prior to conception reduced the prenatal and postnatal viability of their lambs. Correction of iodine deficiency would clearly be of benefit to agriculture.

The epidemiological studies described in Chapters 1–4 indicated the need for animal studies in order to finally prove the relationship between iodine deficiency and brain function. It was clear from the epidemiological evidence that cretinism was associated with severe iodine deficiency (25 per cent of normal intake).

A successful experiment therefore required a severely iodine deficient diet. It proved possible to achieve this in the Merino sheep, an animal that had been studied extensively in Australia following various trace element deficiencies in the soil affecting sheep production. These studies have gone back to the 1930s when cobalt deficiency was first recognized to be a cause of 'coast disease' in sheep. This condition was characterized by loss of appetite and wasting, with death occurring after a few months. Cobalt deficiency prevents the synthesis of the cobalt-containing vitamin B12 in the rumen of the sheep, thus interfering with the metabolism of carbohydrate. The accumulation of pyruvate in the blood causes the loss of appetite and eventual death of the sheep. Coast disease was a major problem for the sheep industry in South and Western Australia, but has now disappeared as a result of correcting the deficiency with the cobalt pellet, first introduced by the CSIRO Division of Animal Nutrition in Adelaide in the 1950s. Subsequent studies have been done on copper deficiency and selenium deficiency.

It was fortunate that scientists experienced in trace element studies were still on the staff when I took charge of the CSIRO Division of Human Nutrition in Adelaide early in 1976. These scientists included a physiologist, Mr Brian Potter, and two chemists, Dr Gordon Jones and Mr Brian Belling, while Dr Richard Smith, a biochemist, assisted in the early discussion. Brian Potter provided excellent leadership of the group over a period of ten years.

Iodine deficiency was known to be a problem with sheep grazing in pastures in many parts of Australia. It was associated, as elsewhere, with poor wool growth, reproductive failure, and goitre in newborn lambs. These areas included Southern Queensland and Northern New South Wales. A series of cereal samples from these areas were analysed by Jones using a particularly sensitive method he had developed. He found several samples with very low iodine content, including maize from the Gatton Agricultural College in Southern Queensland. This maize was selected for feeding the sheep over the next ten years to provide the main component of their diet.

A group of young, proven fertile ewes were then fed the diet which also included pea offal (to provide more fibre), and various trace elements (zinc, calcium, cobalt) to prevent any other deficiency problem. The iodine excretion in the urine was measured, and after some six months had reached very low levels comparable with those observed in areas where endemic cretinism occurred (10–20 μg/day for a 40 kg sheep). After periods of six to twelve months, they were mated with fertile normal rams and became pregnant (Potter *et al.* 1980).

Comparisons were made with a control group of sheep on the same iodine deficient diet but with the addition of an iodine supplement. This was either 2 mg sodium iodide by subcutaneous injection every other, day or later an intramuscular injection of 2 ml iodized oil (960 mg iodine), which lasted for at least three years (Potter *et al.* 1980).

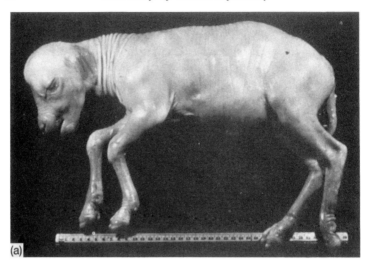

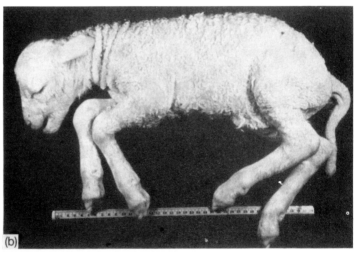

Fig. 5.1. Effect of severe iodine deficiency during pregnancy on lamb development. A 140-day-old lamb fetus (A) was subjected to severe iodine deficiency through feeding the mother an iodine different diet (5-8 μg per day) for 6 months prior to and during pregnancy (full-term 150 days) compared to a control lamb (B) of the same age fed the same diet with the addition of an iodine supplement. The iodine deficient lamb showed absence of wool coat, subluxation of the leg joints, and a dome-like appearance of the head due to skeletal retardation.

Observations were made on the ewes, including thyroid size, the extent of wool growth, and general wellbeing. Large goitres always developed in the iodine deficient ewes. There was some retardation of wool growth with some lack of vitality evident, but otherwise they remained active as in the case of iodine deficient humans.

The fetal lambs were removed before the end of pregnancy by surgical means (hysterotomy) in order to avoid any loss during natural labour and delivery. A retrospective review of the sheep pregnancies showed a 21 per cent loss to the iodine deficient ewes compared to 4 per cent in the controls. This parallels the predisposition to miscarriages and stillbirths of both iodine deficient and hypothyroid human mothers.

The iodine deficient lambs showed a complete absence of wool growth in comparison to the controls (Fig. 5.1). They also showed large goitres, misshapen skulls, and partial dislocation of the leg joints. X-rays of the bones confirmed this and provided evidence of

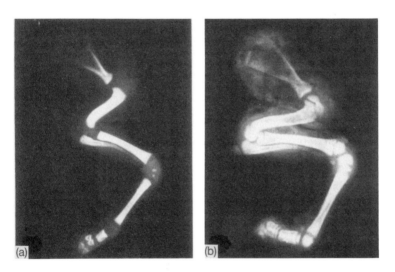

Fig. 5.2. X-rays of the left forelimbs of an iodine deficient (A) and a control (B) fetus of 140 days gestation showing epiphyseal dysgenesis as a result of iodine deficiency. (From Potter *et al.* 1981, with permission.)

delayed ossification of the growing bone centres or epiphyses (Fig. 5.2) (Potter *et al.* 1981). Such a finding is also characteristic of severely hypothyroid children, and I have seen it in severely hypothyroid cretins in Sinjiang Province, China (as described in Chapter 3).

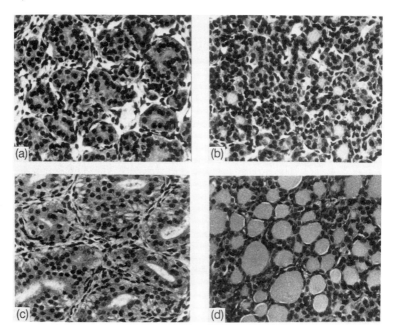

Fig. 5.3. Thyroid tissues of 70-day (A and B) and 140-day (C and D) fetuses. A and C are from iodine deficient and B and D from iodine-replete fetuses. Haematoxylin and eosin stain. (From Potter *et al.* 1981, with permission.)

Observations of the thyroid showed gross hyperplasia of the cells with loss of colloid (Fig. 5.3). Observations of the brains from fetuses removed at various stages during pregnancy revealed lowered brain weight (Fig. 5.4). This was associated with a lessened number of cells as measured by deoxyribonucleic acid (DNA) content (Potter *et al.* 1981). There was a less striking reduction in brain cell size. This finding indicated that there was a slowing in the rate of early nerve cell (neuroblast) multiplication, a process known to occur over the period of 40–80 days' gestation in the sheep. These

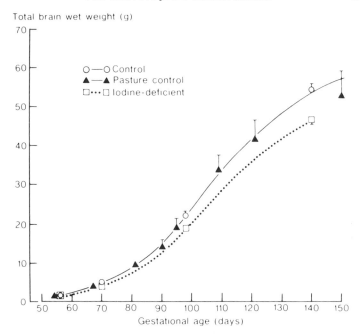

Fig. 5.4. Comparison of brain growth in the fetuses of iodine deficient ewes, ewes fed from pasture, and control ewes fed on an iodine deficient diet supplemented with iodine. (From Potter *et al.* 1981, with permission.) The observed differences can be confidently ascribed to iodine deficiency.

changes were first evident as early as 70 days, or before the end of the first half of pregnancy, the normal gestation period in the sheep being 150 days. The other organs showing significant reduction in weight were the heart and lungs (Fig. 5.5).

Observations under the microscope revealed a denser brain than normal due to a failure of development (arborization) of the normal nerve cell branchings (the axon and the dendrites). This was evident in the cerebral hemisphere and particularly in the cerebellum where retardation in the development of the special Purkinje cells resulted from failure of the normal migration of the granular cells from the external granular layer into the central medulla. (The cerebellum is involved in the smooth coordination of movements. The Purkinje cell acts as a storage cell) (Potter *et al.* 1982).

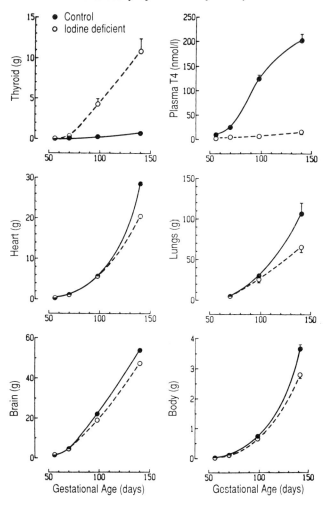

Fig. 5.5. The effect of iodine deficiency on fetal development in the sheep. (From Hetzel *et al.* 1988, with permission.)

The blood levels of thyroid hormones were greatly reduced in both the ewes and the fetuses, associated in each case with grossly reduced thyroid iodine content and gross goitre. At the same time, the level of the pituitary thyroid-stimulating hormone was greatly increased, as would be expected. This hormone causes hyperplasia of the thyroid cells, and goitre, in an attempt to compensate for iodine deficiency by increasing the turnover in the gland (Chapter 1).

That the sheep brain is indeed sensitive to iodine deficiency was indicated by a gross reduction in the level of thyroid hormones in both mother and fetus. Proof that there was a causal relationship between the reduced thyroid hormone secretion and the effects on the brain and other organs was sought through surgical experiments: removal of the thyroid from the fetal lamb at 70 and 98 days' gestation; removal of the maternal thyroid 6 weeks before conception; and a combination of the two procedures. (These surgical procedures depended on the skill of another CSIRO scientist, Dr Graeme McIntosh.)

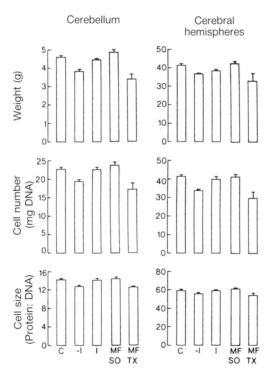

Fig. 5.6. Comparison of brains of sheep fetuses at 140 days' gestation C = control; − I = iodine deficient; I = iodine at 100 days; MFSO = mother + fetus sham-operated; MFTX = mother + fetus thyroidectomized. (From Hetzel 1983, with permission.)

It was found that the fetal thyroidectomy had a similar, but less marked effect, than that of iodine deficiency. Maternal thyroidectomy caused a reduction in fetal brain weight and DNA by mid-gestation (Potter *et al.* 1986). The combination of both produced the same but a more severe effect than that of iodine deficiency, as well as a greater reduction in the level of maternal and fetal blood T_4 levels (McIntosh *et al.* 1983). These effects on the sheep brain are shown in Fig.5.6.

It could be concluded that the effect of the iodine deficiency was mediated through the effects on both maternal and fetal thyroid gland function. This study provided the first experimental evidence of the role of the maternal thyroid in fetal brain development. It has been suspected for many years that reduced thyroid function (hypothyroidism) in the human mother causes mental retardation in the infant and child (Hetzel and Potter. 1983) (Potter *et. al* 1986).

The effects of iodine deficiency on fetal development in sheep can be dramatically reversed by giving the pregnant ewe an injection of iodized oil at 100 days gestation (Fig. 5.6). There is a rapid increase in brain weight and restoration of maternal and fetal thyroid function. Fetal weight is not fully restored however, and the possibility of some residual functional defect in the brain seems likely due to the previous 100 days of severe maternal hypothyroidism. Testing for such a possibility has still to be carried out with studies of behaviour and intellectual performance, but there is evidence from human studies as mentioned above.

There is a difference in the rate of maturation of the brain in the different animal species. For this reason it was decided to pursue studies of iodine deficiency in a monkey (primate) brain to see whether it was as susceptible as the sheep brain. The monkey chosen was the marmoset (*Callithrix jacchus jacchus*) (Fig. 5.7) with a normal habitat in the Amazon jungle in Brazil. These animals require a tropical environment with high humidity and a steady environmental temperature of around 70 °F.

Colonies had been successfully established in England, so we decided to attempt to establish a colony at the CSIRO Division of Human Nutrition in Adelaide, where we had excellent animal facilities. We flew 15 pairs out from the ICI Laboratories at Alderley Park near Manchester (UK) to Australia in the winter of July 1978. The animals flourished thanks to the skilled attention of the CSIRO staff. One of the advantages of studying the marmoset is its ability

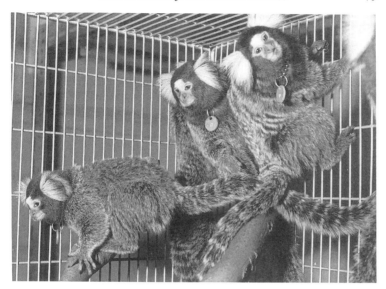

Fig. 5.7. The marmoset provided a valuable opportunity for study of the effects of iodine deficiency on fetal brain development. (Courtesy of Dr G.H. McIntosh.)

to breed in captivity, which is very uncommon with the monkey family as a whole. In fact, 8 out of 10 pregnancies produce twins. They are also readily socialized by frequent handling. Their maximum weight when fully grown is only 500 g so the cost of their food is modest.

The next problem was the iodine deficient diet. One of the staff, Mr Mark Mano, suggested feeding the animals on the iodine-deficient sheep meat. This, with bananas and rat biscuits, provided a soft, high-energy, high-protein diet (Mano *et al.* 1985).

This diet was fed to a group of monogamous animals for a period of twelve months, and to a control group with a sodium iodide supplement. The level of iodine intake was 0.3 µg/day in the iodine deficient group compared with 7.6 µg/day in the controls.

Observable effects of the iodine deficient diet included retardation of growth corresponding to that of the hypothyroid cretin. The fur of the iodine-deficient newborns was rather sparse but otherwise they were not obviously different from the controls.

However, there was an increased thyroid weight with gross reduction of T_4 levels and raised TSH levels in the iodine-deficient neonates. Brain development was shown to be retarded significantly in the progeny of the second iodine-deficient pregnancy, as indicated by reduced weight and DNA in the cerebellum, and increased cell density in the visual cortex with evidence of reduced cell axon and dendrite development, as in the case of the sheep (Mano *et al.* 1987). The findings therefore indicated significant effects of maternal iodine deficiency on primate brain development.

Unfortunately, it has not been possible to continue this research further into studies of the behaviour of these animals, which would be of interest. We hope, however, that colleagues in the Institute of Endocrinology at the Tianjin Medical College, China will be able to do this. In June 1987 a consignment of 15 pairs of marmosets from the CSIRO colony was successfully transported by air to Tianjin. A flourishing colony has now been established in China. This has been made possible by support from the Australia–China Technical Agreement for the Control of Iodine Deficiency Disorders (CIDD) through the Australian International Development Assistance Bureau (AIDAB).

In China, extensive animal studies have been carried out in rats which have been fed a diet identical with that consumed by people living in three severely iodine-deficient areas: Inner Mongolia, Jixian Village (Heilongjiang Province), and Guizhou. In each of these areas severe neurological cretinism is seen, with myxoedematous cretinism also evident in Inner Mongolia.

Rats on these diets show similar brain changes to those described in the sheep: reduced weight and DNA with striking effects on the cerebellum cell architecture, in association with severe hypothyroidism (Li *et al.* 1985). In addition, behavioural and psychometric tests reveal impaired performance under operant conditioning studies (level pressing to avoid a painful stimulus). So far, the full picture of neurological cretinism (paralysis and deafness together with mental defect) has not been seen in these animals. However, only first generation offspring have been observed. Second generation animals are not yet available because of the difficulty of breast feeding by the iodine deficient mothers.

A series of elegant studies in rats has been carried out by Dr Morreale de Escobar and Dr F. Escobar del Rey and their team in Madrid. They have compared pregnant, iodine deficient, rats with rats which had maternal thyroidectomies before pregnancy. There was a reduction in the number of embryos and in their individual body weights following maternal iodine deficiency, with a similar, but more severe effect following maternal thyroidectomy (Morreale de Escobar *et al.* 1986). Measurements of the pyramidal tract in the visual cortex showed retardation following maternal iodine deficiency similar to that observed following maternal thyroidectomy. Recovery from the effect required early iodine replacement within the first 10 days which underlines the importance of early correction of iodine deficiency, preferably before pregnancy.

These effects confirm the importance of maternal thyroid function for embryonic development. Subsequent studies in the rat have revealed evidence of transfer of the maternal thyroid hormone across the placental barrier early in pregnancy (Obregon *et al.* 1984).

Conclusion

We may conclude from our review of these animal studies that a sufficient supply of iodine is essential for normal growth and development in a variety of animal species including the primate. A deficiency of iodine leads to a reduction in the supply of both maternal and fetal thyroid hormones which are essential for normal brain development. Indeed, the importance of the maternal thyroid hormone supply, although implicated by human studies for some years, has now been proved by these animal studies. Finally, it has been demonstrated recently that there is transfer of maternal thyroid hormones across the placenta early in pregnancy in the rat. This is probably also true of other species and of the human, as suggested by indirect evidence in man.

Bibliography

Hetzel, B.S. (1983). Iodine deficiency disorders (IDD) and their eradication. *Lancet* **2**, 1126–29.
—— and Potter, B.J. (1983). Iodine deficiency and the role of thyroid hormones in brain development. In *Neurobiology of the trace elements* (eds. I. Dreosti and R.M. Smith), pp. 83–133. Humana Press, New Jersey.
Hetzel, B.S., Potter, B.J., and Dulberg E.M. (1988). The iodine deficiency disorders: nature, pathogenesis and epidemiology. *World Review of Nutrition and Dietetics* (in the press).

Li J., Wang X., Yan Y., Want K., Qin D., Xin Z., and Wei J. (1985) The effects of a severely iodine deficient diet derived from an endemic area on fetal brain development in the rat: observations in the first generation. *Neuropathology and Applied Neurobiology* **12** 261–76.

McIntosh, G. H., Potter, B. J., Mano, M. T., Hua, C. H., Cragg, B. G., and Hetzel, B. S. (1983). The effect of maternal and fetal thyroidectomy on fetal brain development in the sheep. *Neuropathology and Applied Neurobiology* **9**, 215–23.

Mano, M. T., Potter, B. J., Belling, G. B., and Hetzel, B. S. (1985). Low-iodine diet for the production of severe I deficiency in marmosets (*Callithrix jacchus jacchus*). *British Journal of Nutrition* **54**, 367–72.

Mano, M. T., Potter, B. J., Belling, G. B., Chavadej, J., and Hetzel, B. S. (1987). Fetal brain development in response to iodine deficiency in a primate model (*Callithrix jacchus jacchus*). *Journal of the Neurological Sciences* **79**, 287–300.

Morreale de Escobar, G., Escobar del Rey, F., Obregon, M. J., and Ruiz-Marcos, A. (1986). The hypothyroid rat. In *Iodine deficiency disorders and congenital hypothyroidism* (eds. G. Medeiros-Neto, R. M. B., Maciel, and A. Halpern), pp. 52–64. Ache, São Paulo, Brazil.

Obregon, M. J., Santisteban, P., Rodiguez-pena, A., Pascual, A., Cartagena, P., Ruiz-Marcos, A., Lamas, L., Escobar del Rey, F., and Morreale de Escobar, G. (1984). Cerebral hypothyroidism in rats with adult-onset iodine deficiency. *Endocrinology* **115**, 614–24.

Potter, B. J., McIntosh, G. H., and Hetzel, B. S. (1981). The effect of iodine deficiency on fetal brain development in sheep, In *Fetal brain disorders: recent approaches to the problem of mental deficiency* (eds. B. S. Hetzel, and R. M. Smith) pp. 119–48. Elsevier, Amsterdam.

Potter, B. J., Jones, G. B., Buckley, R. A., Belling, G. B., McIntosh, G. H., and Hetzel, B. S. (1980). Production of severe iodine deficiency in sheep using a prepared low-iodine diet. *Australian Journal of Biological Sciences* **33**, 53–61.

Potter, B. J., Mano, M. T., Belling, G. B., McIntosh, G. H., Hua, C., Cragg, B. G., Marshall, J., Wellby, M. L., and Hetzel, B. S, (1982). Retarded fetal brain development resulting from severe dietary iodine deficiency in sheep. *Neuropathology and Applied Neurobiology* **8**, 303–13.

Potter, B. J., McIntosh, G. H., Mano, M. T., Chavadej, J., Hua, C. H., Cragg, B. G., and Hetzel, B. S. (1986). The effect of maternal thyroidectomy prior to conception on fetal brain development in sheep. *Acta Endocrinologica* **112**, 93–9.

Further reading

Hetzel, B. S. and Maberly, G. F. (1985). Iodine. In *Trace elements in human and animal nutrition* (ed. W. Mertz), 5th edn, Vol. 2, pp. 139–208. Academic Press, New York.

6

The spectrum of iodine deficiency disorders

The last four chapters have discussed the effects of iodine deficiency in a number of different settings, particularly Alpine Europe and Papua New Guinea, and in animals as well as in humans. This chapter provides a comprehensive overview of these effects and puts forward the all-inclusive concept of iodine deficiency disorders (IDD).

This term was suggested in 1983 to denote all the effects of iodine

Table 6.1 *The spectrum of iodine deficiency disorders (IDD)*

Fetus	Abortions
	Stillbirths
	Congenital anomalies
	Increased perinatal mortality
	Increased infant mortality

	Neurological cretinism—mental deficiency
	        deaf mutism
	        spastic diplegia
	        squint

	Myxoedematous cretinism—dwarfism mental deficiency
	Psychomotor defects
Neonate	Neonatal goitre
	Neonatal hypothyroidism
Child and adolescent	Goitre
	Juvenile hypothyroidism
	Impaired mental function
	Retarded physical development
Adult	Goitre with its complications
	Hypothyroidism
	Impaired mental function
	Iodine induced hyperthyroidism

From Hetzel (1987), with permission.

deficiency on growth and development (Hetzel 1983). In the past, the term 'goitre' has been used. Goitre is indeed the obvious and familiar feature, but our knowledge has greatly expanded in the last 25 years, so that it is not surprising that a new term is needed. The term IDD has in fact now been generally adopted in the field of international nutrition and health. This reconceptualization of the problem—'packaged' in the acronym IDD—has been one factor in securing much more attention to the problem.

A comprehensive list of the iodine deficiency disorders is shown in Table 6.1. It is convenient to list and discuss them by reference to the stage of development in which they originate. By definition all these conditions can be prevented by correction of the deficiency. Nearly all of them can be effectively treated by correction of the deficiency. The exceptions are the fetal disorders. Let us now review IDD in detail by reference to the four stages of life in which it occurs.

Iodine deficiency in the fetus

In iodine deficient areas there is an increased rate of spontaneous abortions and stillbirths in humans which can be reduced by correction of the deficiency. Similar benefits follow thyroid treatment in the pregnant mother who is hypothyroid (McMichael *et al.* 1980).

An increased rate of stillbirths has also been observed in iodine deficient sheep. In iodine deficient pastures, lamb losses can be reduced by correction of the deficiency. Similar observations have been made with goats. This effect can be produced experimentally with hypothyroidism. For example, studies in hypothyroid guinea pigs (produced by surgical removal of the thyroid) reveal a three- to four-fold increase in abortions and stillbirths which can be virtually eliminated by replacement therapy with thyroxine during pregnancy (McMichael *et al.* 1980).

In the iodine deficient rat, there is both a smaller number of embryos and a reduced size of embryo produced. Similar changes of a more severe degree follow maternal thyroidectomy in the rat. (See Chapter 5.)

Data from Zaire and Papua New Guinea indicate an increase in stillbirths and infant mortality. The results of a controlled trial in Zaire of iodized oil injections given in the latter half of pregnancy, alternately with a control injection, are shown in Table 6.2. There is

Table 6.2 *Effect of injection of iodized oil given during pregnancy in Zaire**

	Not treated	Treated
Birth weight (g)	2634 ± 552	2837 ± 542 +
	(98)	(112)
Perinatal mortality per 1000	188	98 +
	(123)	(129)
Infant mortality per 1000	250	167 +
	(263)	(252)
Development quotient	104 ± 24	115 ± 16 +
	(66)	(72)

Number of subjects in brackets
+ Difference significant
Modified from Thilly (1981), with permission.

a substantial fall in perinatal and infant mortality with improved birth weight. Low birth weight is generally associated with a higher rate of congenital anomalies and higher risk through childhood. Such a high risk throughout childhood was shown in the follow-up of the controlled trial with iodized oil in the Western Highlands of New Guinea cited in Chapter 4.

Recent evidence indicates that the effects of iodine deficiency on the fetus, including abortion, stillbirth, congenital anomalies, and the varying manifestations of cretinism, probably arise from the lowered level of blood T_4 in the iodine deficient mother. The more severe the reduction in the level of maternal T_4, the greater the threat to the integrity of the fetus. The data from Papua New Guinea cited in Chapter 4 clearly support this concept. It is also supported by animal data in the case of abortions and stillbirths.

All these findings indicate the major impact of iodine deficiency on child survival.

Iodine deficiency in the neonate

Neonatal goitre was once commonly seen in iodine deficient areas. It is still seen in sheep grazing on iodine deficient pastures, and is a cause of loss of lambs. It can be reduced by iodine supplementation. In humans, a reduction in neonatal goitre was described in Austria in 1954 following use of potassium iodide from the fourth month of pregnancy. There was a reduction of goitre rate in the newborn from 47 per cent to 5 per cent in two years (Kopf 1954).

Neonatal hypothyroidism is a well-recognized cause of mental defect. This is due to the fact that the development of the brain is dependent on an adequate supply of thyroxine. Only about one third of normal brain development occurs before birth and the other two-thirds is completed in the first two years of life. Hence a normal level of thyroxine is all-important both during and after pregnancy.

In many countries every newborn child is tested for the level of blood thyroxine (usually taken from a prick in the heel at the 4th and 5th day of life). If the level is found to be low, indicating a lowered state of thyroid gland function, further check is made. If confirmed, replacement treatment with daily tablets of thyroxine is begun immediately. The results have been evaluated in several countries and are generally excellent, provided treatment is given within the first month of life. In Western countries, the incidence of such an abnormality runs at 1 per 3500 live births due to either the absence of the thyroid, an abnormal fetal position (ectopia), or a defect in the 'biochemical machinery' required to produce thyroxine (called a biosynthetic defect). In iodine deficient environments, however,

Table 6.3 *Iodine deficiency and incidence of neonatal chemical hypothyroidism (NCH)*

Area of study	Goitre prevalence	Cretinism prevalence	Urinary iodine Follis group[++]	Incidence of NCH (per 1000 births)
Bhutan	60%	2–13%	V	115
Deoria	80%	3–5%	V	133
Gorakhpur	70%	0–4%	V	85
Gonda	60%	0–4%	V	75
Kathmandu (Nepal)[+]	NA	NA	II	15
Delhi	29%	nil	II	6
Kerala	1.3%	nil	NA	1

[+] Ongoing partially successful iodized salt prophylaxis
[++] Group II: None with urinary iodines less than 25 $\mu g/g$ creatinine; Group V: more than 50% with less than 25 $\mu g/g$.
NA Not available

From Kochupillai and Pandav (1987), with permission.

observations of blood taken from the umbilical vein (in the umbilical cord) just after birth reveal a much higher rate of neonatal hypothyroidism—up to 10 per cent in Zaire and 5-10 per cent in Northern India and Nepal (Table 6.3).

Table 6.3 presents the results of screening 20 000 newborns in India, Nepal, and Bhutan. Neonatal chemical hypothyroidism was defined by a thyroxine level lower than 3 μg/dl and a thyroid-stimulating hormone level greater than 50 μl/ml. It was correlated with severity of iodine deficiency as assessed by prevalence of goitre, prevalence of cretinism, and level of iodine in the urine.

In the most severely deficient environments, where more than 50 per cent had urinary iodine below 25 μg per gram creatinine (25 per cent of normal intake), the incidence of neonatal hypothyroidism was 75-115 per thousand births. By contrast in Delhi where only mild iodine deficiency was present with low prevalence of goitre and no cretinism, the incidence dropped to 6 per thousand. In control areas without goitre, the level was only one per thousand.

In Zaire, where similar observations have been made, hypothyroidism persists into infancy and childhood, with resultant physical and mental retardation (Thilly *et al.* 1986).

In India these chemical observations have been extended to studies of the IQs and hearing of school children (Kochupillai and Pandav 1987). It has been shown that there is a marked reduction in IQ scores in villages with a high rate of (chemical) hypothyroidism. Nerve deafness is much more common, and there is evidence of lowered growth hormone levels in the blood.

These observations indicate a much greater risk of mental defect than is indicated by the presence of cretinism. They indicate the major impact of iodine deficiency on child development.

A very convenient and cheap method for assessment of severity of iodine deficiency, provided a laboratory is available, is being gradually established in India, China, and Indonesia. Samples of cord blood which have been spread on specially prepared filter paper (Whatman No. 3) are sent through the post to the biochemistry laboratory, where radioimmunoassay for T_4 and TSH is carried out. The equipment is complex and expensive but automated so that large numbers of samples can be processed.

So far it is not possible, due to inadequacy of manpower and money, to diagnose and treat infants in most Third World countries. Hence the overwhelming importance of prevention. An injection of

480 mg of iodine in oil given to a hypothyroid mother during pregnancy will provide iodine through her breast milk for two to three years. Alternatively, a small dose of the oil given to the infant will provide the iodine for normal thyroid function and brain development. Observations on neonatal hypothyroidism in Europe are discussed in Chapter 10.

Iodine deficiency in infancy and childhood

Iodine deficiency in children is characteristically associated with goitre. The classification of goitre has now been standardized by the World Health Organization and is discussed in Chapter 8. The rate increases with age, reaching a maximum with adolescence. Girls have a higher prevalence than boys. Observations of goitre rates in schoolchildren over the period 8–14 years provides a convenient indication of community prevalence. The availability of children in schools is a great advantage in providing access to a population. Collections of casual samples of urine can also be conveniently carried out.

The prevention and control of goitre in schoolchildren was first demonstrated by Marine and Kimball in Akron, Ohio, in 1917. The results of these studies have been discussed in Chapter 1. However, Marine and Kimball recognized in 1921 that goitre was only part of IDD: 'The prevention of goitre means vastly more than cervical [neck] deformities. It means in addition, the prevention of those forms of physical and mental degeneration such as cretinism, mutism, and idiocy which are dependent on thyroid insufficiency. Further it would prevent the development of thyroid adenomas which are an integral and essential part of endemic goitre in man and due to the same stimulus.'

Recent studies in children living in iodine deficient areas from a number of countries indicate impaired school performance and IQs in comparison with matched groups from non-iodine-deficient areas. These studies are difficult to set up because of the problem of the control group. There are many possible causes for impaired school performance and impaired performance on an IQ test which make difficult the interpretation of any difference that might be observed. The iodine deficient area is likely to be more remote, suffer more social deprivation, and have a disadvantage in school facilities, a lower socioeconomic status, and poorer general nutrition. All such factors have to be taken into account, apart from the problem of adapting tests developed in Western countries for use in Third World countries (Stanbury 1987).

Initially, studies of psychomotor development as indicated by tests of motor coordination revealed differences that could be regarded as, to a large extent, independent of educational status. In Papua New Guinea, as discussed in Chapter 4, differences in bi-manual dexterity were revealed by threading beads and putting pegs into a pegboard. These differences have been significantly related to the level of maternal thyroxine at the time of pregnancy and have persisted up to the age of 10–12 years. Differences of motor coordi-nation have also been observed in Indonesia. The differences in psychomotor development became apparent only after the age of two-and-a-half years. Similar data are now becoming available from China.

Furthermore, Bleichrodt and colleagues (1987) using a wide range of psychological tests have shown that the mental development of children from iodine deficient areas lags behind that of children from non-iodine-deficient areas.

The next question is whether these differences can be affected by correction of the deficiency. In a pioneering study initiated in Ecuador from 1966 to 1986 by Fierro-Benitez and colleagues, the long-term effects of iodized oil injections were assessed by compa-rison of two Highland villages. One (Tocachi) was treated, the other (La Esperanza) was used as a control. Particular attention was paid to 128 children aged 8–15, whose mothers had received iodized oil prior to the second trimester of pregnancy, and to a matched control group of 293 of similar age. All children were examined at birth and at key stages in their development. Women in Tocachi were injected or re-injected in 1970, 1974, and 1978. Assessments in 1973, 1978, and 1981 revealed the following.

Scholastic achievement was better in the children of treated mothers when measured in terms of school year reached for age, school drop-out rate, failure rate, years repeated, and school marks. There was no difference between the two groups by certain tests (Terman–Merrill, Wechsler scale, or Goodenough). Both groups were impaired in school performance, in reading, writing, and mathematics, but more notably the children of untreated mothers.

The results indicate the significant role of iodine deficiency, but other factors were also important in the school performance of these

Ecuadorean children, such as social deprivation and nutrition.

In 1982 the results were reported of a controlled trial carried out with oral iodized oil in a small Highland village (Tiquipaya) 2645 metres above sea level in Bolivia (Bautista *et al.* 1982). The children did not show clinical evidence of protein caloric malnutrition. The mean serum PBI had been low (1.7 μg/dl) in 1970. Of 408 children examined, 100 boys and 100 girls were chosen for further study in the age group 5½–12 years, all with some degree of thyroid enlargement. Goitre size was estimated using the standard methods and IQ was measured with the Stanford Binet in Spanish, using the short form test. The Bender Gestalt was also used.

Each child in the treatment group received an oral dose of 1.0 ml iodized oil (475 mg iodine) while children in the second group received 1.0 ml of a non-iodine containing mineral oil of a similar brown colour. Subsequent assessment was double blind. On follow-up 22 months later, the urinary iodine had increased and goitre size had decreased in both groups. This reflected 'contamination' of the village environment with iodine due probably to urine excretion by those who had received the iodized oil injections. There were no differences between the two treatment groups in growth rate or in the performance with the tests. However, improvement in IQ could be demonstrated in all children, regardless of their group, who showed significant reduction of goitre. This was particularly so in girls. It was concluded that correction of iodine deficiency may improve the mental performance of school age children, but that a bigger dose should be given.

These results further emphasize the importance of adequate iodine intake for normal child development.

Iodine deficiency in the adult

The most common effect of iodine deficiency in adults is goitre. Characteristically there is an absence of classical clinical hypo-thyroidism in adults with endemic goitre. However, laboratory evidence of hypothyroidism with reduced T_4 levels is common. This is often accompanied by normal T_3 levels and raised TSH levels.

Iodine administration in the form of iodized salt, bread, or oil has been demonstrated to be effective in the prevention of goitre in adults. It may also reduce existing goitre in adults. This is particularly true of iodized oil injections. A rise in circulating thyroxine can be demonstrated in adult subjects following iodization (Fig. 4.9).

In Northern India a high degree of apathy has been noted in populations living in iodine deficient areas. (This may even affect domestic animals such as dogs!) It is apparent that reduced mental function is widely prevalent in iodine deficient communities with effects on initiative and decision-making. This means that iodine deficiency is a major block to human and social development.

The social benefits of iodization have been well described by the observations of Professor Li and his group (1987). In the north-east Chinese village of Jixian in the Heilongjiang Province in 1978, there were 1313 people with a goitre rate of 65 per cent and 11.4 per cent cretins. The cretins included many severe cases, which caused the village to be known locally as 'the village of idiots'. The economic development of the village was retarded— for example, no truck driver or teacher was available. Girls from other villages did not want to marry and live in village. The intelligence of the student population was known to be low: children aged 10 had a mental development equivalent to those aged 7.

Iodized salt was introduced in 1978, after which the goitre rate dropped to 4 per cent by 1982. No cretins had been born since 1978. The attitude of the people had changed greatly; they were much more positive in their approach to life in contrast to their attitude before iodization. The average income had increased from 43 yuan per head in 1981 to 223 yuan in 1982 and 414 yuan in 1984, which was higher than the average income per capita in the district. In 1983, cereals were exported for the first time. Before iodization, no family had a radio, but in 1982 55 families had a TV set. From 1978 to 1982, 44 girls came from other villages to marry boys in Jixian. Seven men had joined the People's Liberation Army whereas before there had been no enlistments because of rejection for goitre.

Iodine-induced hyperthyroidism

This condition is a complication of the correction of iodine deficiency occurring mainly in those over the age of 45 with long-standing deficiency. As it can be completely prevented by earlier correction, it belongs to IDD. It is discussed in Chapter 7.

A quantitative estimate of IDD in populations

This review has described a spectrum of effects spread through the various stages of life. It would be a great advantage to have some quantitative estimates of the dimension of these disorders, in order to more readily assess the impact of iodine deficiency on a population, and so indicate the benefits that could be expected from prevention and control.

The usual feature of IDD which has been estimated in a population has been the prevalence of goitre at the various gradations of severity (grade 1, 2, 3). The most commonly studied group has been schoolchildren. Extensive data are now available from many countries. The relation between the goitre rate in schoolchildren and the total goitre rate in the community has been examined by Dr Eric Dulberg in specific countries where both categories of data are available, such as Bhutan and Indonesia. From these data a functional relationship has been derived, with which the goitre rate in children can be transformed into the goitre rate for the whole population (Dulberg 1985; Clugston *et al.* 1987).

Total goitre rate and cretinism

The next question that arises is whether it is possible to derive from the goitre rate of a community quantitative estimates of some of the other iodine deficiency disorders such as cretinism. Fodéré in 1792 noted that the mothers of cretins were nearly always goitrous though not usually themselves cretins. Epidemiological data from Papua New Guinea indicate that the risk of cretinism in the child increases with the goitre rate in the mother. In the light of the earlier discussion in this chapter relating cretinism to the level of maternal T_4, this can be explained by the progressive lowering of the serum T_4 in mothers.

There are data from a number of countries indicating the close relationship between cretinism, and the goitre rate of the community. These include Papua New Guinea, Peru, Argentina, and Switzerland. A detailed analysis of the relationship has been carried out using recent data from Zaire and Ecuador (Dulberg 1985; Clugston *et al* 1987). There have also been a number of individual community surveys from various countries in Asia. From these

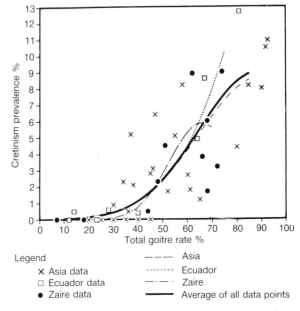

Fig. 6.1. Relationship between total goitre rate and cretinism prevalence based on three sets of community survey data: from Asia, Ecuador, and Zaire. (From Clugston *et al.* 1987, with permission.)

three categories of data three independent estimates of the functional relationship have been made (Dulberg 1985; Clugston *et al.* 1987). These have been found to be very close throughout virtually the range of goitre prevalence (Fig. 6.1). Only at the upper end of the goitre range (goitre rates over 70 per cent) where there are insufficient data available, do the three functions diverge from each other. Hence a general equation has been generated to express the relation between goitre and cretinism based on the combined three sets of data. This equation has been used to generate estimates of cretinism prevalence in the eight South-east Asian countries of the WHO region.

Attempts have also been made to quantitate 'cretinoids', those sufferers of the less severe effects of iodine deficiency described earlier in this chapter. Because of the variety of manifestations and the difficulty of measurement criteria which encompass mental, psychomotor, and other neurological defects, quantitative analyses are very difficult. However, it can be assumed that the model for these relationships is similar to that of cretinism based on the level of maternal T_4 so that a 'constant multiplier' can be postulated. Three different iodine-deficiency-related states have been considered: hearing loss, motor defect, and reduced mental performance.

Regarding the first category of cretinoids, a thorough field study in the Sengi community in Central Java revealed a goitre rate of 85 per cent and a cretin rate of 8.2 per cent. Formal audiometry revealed another 4.2 per cent of individuals with bilateral perceptive hearing loss with some other mild mental or motor defect. Hence inclusion of this group increases the cretinism prevalence rate by 50 per cent.

Study of the age of walking in the same community revealed that an inability to walk at the age of two years was less prevalent in children whose mothers received iodized oil in pregnancy. Such a defect had been previously observed by Pharoah in New Guinea (Chapter 4).

The 'multiplier' estimated from these two additional groups was 2.75.

Table 6.4 *Estimated populations at risk, and prevalence of endemic goitre in eight countries of the WHO South-east Asian region (Numbers in thousands)*

Country	Total Pop.	Population at risk (TGR > 10%)		Endemic goitre prevalence	
		Number	%	Number	%
Bangladesh	97 438	37 150	38.1	10 225	10.5
Bhutan	1446	1446	100.	946	65.4
Burma	39 920	14 545	36.5	5694	14.3
India	746 010	149 588	20.0	54 318	7.3
Indonesia	161 003	29 773	18.5	9759	6.1
Nepal	16 386	15 099	92.0	7555	46.1
Sri Lanka	16 099	10 565	65.6	3112	19.3
Thailand	52 709	20 439	38.8	7740	14.7
TOTAL	1131 011	278 605	24.6	99 349	8.8

Note: TGR = Total Goitre Rate (prevalence).
Percentages shown are percentages of total population.
From *UN Demographic Yearbook* (1981/2) and Clugston *et al.* (1987), with permission.

Regarding the second category, psychomotor tests, there was a definite excess of individuals in a iodine deficient village in Indonesia, Gowok compared to an non-iodine-deficient village (Longjong). The estimated multiplier from the difference was 3.15.

Data on intellectual development was obtained in two villages in Ecuador with an average goitre rate of 74 per cent, and a 7 per cent prevalence of cretinism. IQ scores in children of mothers given iodized oil prior to conception were compared with children born to non-injected mothers. There was a definite shift to lower scores in the children of the untreated mothers. This difference yielded a multiplier of 3.0.

It was assumed (conservatively) that the same children would be affected by each of the three manifestations of milder IDD related

Table 6.5 *Estimated IDD prevalence in eight IDD affected countries of the WHO South-east Asian region*

Country	Endemic goitre		Endemic cretinism (A)		Milder mental/ motor handicap (B)*		Total IDD handicap (A + B)	
	No.	%	No.	%	No.	%	No.	%
Bangladesh	10 225	10.5	354	0.36	1062	1.08	1416	1.44
Bhutan	946	65.4	81	5.58	242	16.73	323	22.31
Burma	5694	14.3	305	0.76	914	2.29	1219	3.05
India	54 318	7.3	2209	0.30	6626	0.89	8835	1.19
Indonesia	9759	6.1	427	0.27	1280	0.81	1707	1.08
Nepal	7555	46.1	526	3.21	1578	9.63	2104	12.84
Sri Lanka	3112	19.3	79	0.49	236	1.46	315	1.95
Thailand	7740	14.7	402	0.76	1206	2.29	1608	3.05
TOTAL	99 349	8.8	4383	0.39	13 144	1.16	17 527	1.55

Note: Percentages shown are percentages of total population.

* Milder mental, motor, and other developmental handicap (deficit or delay): includes persons with multiple or single cretinous features short of full cretinism as identifiable in a typical field study setting. This includes an estimated proportion of persons, in endemic areas, who score below the mean of mental or motor ability tests *in excess* of the proportion of persons who score below the mean in a comparable but non-endemic area.

From WHO, and for Total Population, *UN Demographic Yearbook* (1981/1982), and Clugston *et al.* (1987), with permission.

brain damage. Hence a factor of 3 was used for the total estimate of IDD–attributed lesser defects in addition to cretinism.

Based on the goitre prevalence in the eight countries of the WHO South-east Asian region (Table 6.4), Dulberg has tabulated the estimates for the IDD related brain defects (Table 6.5).

These estimates indicate significant IDD prevalence. Of the total goitrous population of nearly 100 million in these eight countries, 1.55 per cent (in excess of 17 million) have IDD related handicap, including more than 4 million cretins. I believe this order of magnitude is a reasonable estimate of the problem of IDD in the South-east Asian region. A more precise estimate can be achieved as data become available.

Total goitre rate, stillbirths, and neonatal deaths

The possibility of relating goitre rate to fetal effects of severe iodine deficiency (stillbirths and neonatal deaths) has also been explored by Dulberg (1985). The data used was derived from four reported

Table 6.6 *Estimated number and rate of stillbirths and neonatal deaths, and their sum (total late reproductive loss) attributable to iodine deficiency in eight countries of the WHO South-east Asian region.*

Country	Stillbirths		Neonatal deaths		Total late reproductive loss	
	No.*	Rate**	No.*	Rate**	No.*	Rate**
Bangladesh	10.5	2.3	9.6	2.1	20.1	4.4
Bhutan	2.3	36.6	2.1	33.6	4.4	70.2
Burma	7.6	5.0	7.0	4.5	14.6	9.5
India	47.4	1.9	43.5	1.8	90.9	3.7
Indonesia	9.2	1.7	8.5	1.6	17.7	3.3
Nepal	15.0	21.0	13.8	19.3	28.8	40.3
Sri Lanka	1.4	3.1	1.3	2.8	2.7	5.9
Thailand	8.4	4.9	7.7	4.5	16.1	9.4
TOTAL	101.8	2.6	93.5	2.4	195.3	5.0

* Number in thousands
** Rate expressed as number per 1000 live births

From Clugston *et al.* (1987), with permission.

controlled trials using iodized oil in severely iodine deficient communities (Ecuador, Papua New Guinea, Peru, and Zaire). In each case, fewer stillbirths and neonatal deaths were reported in the groups receiving iodized oil (Clugston *et al.* 1987).

In view of the importance of maternal T_4 levels to these effects as in the case of cretinism, it seems reasonable to expect a similar relationship to that between cretinism and goitre rates.

Using these data, internally consistent indices have been derived which can be used to calculate stillbirths and neonatal deaths in whole populations of the South-east Asian countries. Table 6.6 presents a vivid picture of the impact of iodine deficiency in these eight countries. More data are needed to confirm these estimates in these and other regions, particularly Africa. However, it is quite clear that IDD represents a major threat to the fetus.

Future research

Attempts are now being made to assess the socioeconomic impact of IDD. Productivity as indicated by farm income, school performance, and other community indicators needs to be measured before and after the introduction of IDD control measures. This is not easy because of the difficulty of separating the effects of an IDD control programme from other factors in development and productivity such as capital in-flow and improvements in farm technology and transportation.

The effect of correction of iodine deficiency in farm animals is a significant socioeconomic benefit which could be more readily measured.

Conclusion

Iodine deficiency disorders (IDD) include:

(1) goitre at all ages;
(2) endemic cretinism, characterized most commonly by mental deficiency, deaf mutism, spastic diplegia, and lesser degrees of neurological defect related to fetal iodine deficiency;
(3) impaired mental function in children and adults, associated with reduced levels of circulating thyroxine;
(4) increased stillbirths and infant mortality.

Adequate evidence is now available, both from controlled trials and successful iodization programmes, that IDD can be prevented by correction of the deficiency. Effects on child survival and development are particularly important.

The social impact of IDD is very much due to depressing effects on mental and physical energy. Prevention has resulted in improved quality of life, productivity of adults, and school performance of children.

A model derived from extensive epidemiological data linking goitre and cretinism enables calculations of the numbers suffering from various forms of IDD. These data, from South-east Asia, reveal massive effects which make prevention and control of IDD an urgent priority.

This review represents a synthesis of the results of study of the problem of iodine deficiency over the last 40 years. A more comprehensive review of human, animal, and epidemiological data has been provided elsewhere (Hetzel *et al.* 1988).

In view of the feasibility of the prevention and control of IDD, demonstrated in a number of controlled trials and studies following IDD control programmes, an opportunity exists for a spectacular success in international health and nutrition.

Bibliography

Bautista, A., Barker, P.A., Dunn, J.T., Sanchez, M., and Kaiser, D.L. (1982). The effects of oral iodized oil on intelligence, thyroid status, and somatic growth in school-age children from an area of endemic goitre. *American Journal Clinical Nutrition* 35, 127-34.

Bleichrodt, N., Garcia, I., Rubio, C., Morreale de Escobar, G., and Escobar Del Rey, F. (1987). Developmental disorders associated with severe iodine deficiency. In *The prevention and control of iodine deficiency disorders* (eds. B.S. Hetzel, J.T. Dunn and J.B. Stanbury) pp. 65-84. Elsevier, Amsterdam.

Clugston, G.A., Dulberg, E.M., Pandav, C.S., and Tilden, R.L. (1987). Iodine deficiency disorders in South East Asia. In *The prevention and control of iodine deficiency disorders* (eds. B.S. Hetzel, J.T. Dunn, and J.B. Stanbury) pp. 273-308. Elsevier, Amsterdam.

Dulberg, E.M. (1985). A model for predicting the prevalence of developmental iodine deficiency disorders from goitre data: a preliminary report. *IDD Newsletter* 1(1), 6.

Fierro-Renoy, F., and Estrella, E. (1986). Long-term effect of correction of iodine deficiency on psychomotor and intellectual development. In *Towards the eradication of endemic goiter, cretinism and iodine deficiency* (eds. J.T. Dunn, E. Pretell, Daza, and F.E. Viteri) pp. 182–200. PAHO, Washington.

Fodére, M. (1792). Essai sur le goitre et le crétinege. De l'Imprimeur Royale.

Hetzel, B.S. (1983). Iodine deficiency disorders (IDD) and their eradication. *Lancet* **2**, 1126–9.

—— (1987). An overview of the prevention and control of iodine deficiency disorders. In The *prevention and control of iodine deficiency disorders* (eds. B.S. Hetzel, J.T. Dunn, and J.B. Stanbury) pp. 7–31. Elsevier, Amsterdam.

Hetzel, B.S., Potter, B.J., and Dulberg, E.M. (1988). The iodine deficiency disorders: nature, pathogenesis and epidemiology. *World Review of Nutrition and Dietetics*, in the press.

Kochupillai, N. and Pandav, C.S. (1987). Neonatal chemical hypothyroidism in iodine deficient environments. In *The prevention and control of iodine deficiency disorders* (eds. B.S. Hetzel, J.T. Dunn, and J.B. Stanbury) pp. 85–93. Elsevier, Amsterdam.

Kopf, H. (1954). *Wien. klin. Wschr,* **66**, 96.

Lancet editorial. (1983). From endemic goitre to iodine deficiency disorders. *Lancet* **2**, 1121–2.

Li, J.Q. and Wang, X. (1987). Jixian: A success story in IDD control. *IDD Newsletter* **3** (1), 4–5.

Marine, D. and Kimball, O.P. (1921). The prevention of simple goitre in man. *Journal of the American Medical Association* **77**, 1068–72.

McMichael, A.J., Potter, J.D., and Hetzel, B.S. (1980). Iodine deficiency, thyroid function, and reproductive failure. In *Endemic goiter and endemic cretinism* (eds. J.B. Stanbury and B.S. Hetzel) pp. 445–60. Wiley, New York.

Stanbury, J.B. (1987). The iodine deficiency disorders: introduction and general aspects. In *The prevention and control of iodine deficiency disorders* (eds. B.S. Hetzel, J.T. Dunn, and J.B. Stanbury) pp. 35–48. Elsevier, Amsterdam.

Thilly, C.H., Bourdoux, P.P., Vanderpas, J.B., Swennen, B.A., Deckx, H.P., Luvivila, G.K., and Delange, F.M. (1986). Neonatal and juvenile hypothyroidism in Central Africa. In: Iodine deficiency disorders and congenital hypothyroidism (eds. G. Medeiros-Neto, R.M.B. Maciel, and A. Halpern) pp. 26–33. Ache, Brazil.

Further reading

Hetzel, B. S, Dunn, J. T., and Stanbury, J. B. (eds.) (1987). *The prevention and control of iodine deficiency disorders*. Elsevier, Amsterdam.

Hetzel, B. S., Potter, B. J., and Dulberg, E. M. (1988). The iodine deficiency disorders: nature, pathogenesis and epidemiology. *World Review of Nutrition and Dietetics*, in the press.

Stanbury, J. B. and Hetzel, B. S. (eds.) (1980). *Endemic goiter and endemic cretinism: iodine nutrition in health and disease*. Wiley, New York.

PART II

Preventing and controlling iodine deficiency disorders

7

The correction of iodine deficiency

We shall now consider in detail the prevention and control of goitre and IDD through iodine supplementation. Iodized salt, iodized oil, iodized bread, and iodized water will be reviewed.

The main global sources of iodine are the USA, Japan, and Chile. China is at present totally dependent on Japan for its iodine supplies, as is Indonesia. This means that purchase of iodine involves scarce supplies of foreign exchange so that the economic costs are significant.

Iodine is available from oil, brine, and natural gas wells. A special process is available for extraction which means that it might be produced by countries with an oil industry. The oil should be free of sulphur for this purpose.

Iodized salt

There are two forms of iodine which can be used to iodize salt: 'iodide' as in 'iodized salt', and 'iodate' as in 'iodated salt'. Iodate is less soluble and more stable than iodide and is therefore preferred for tropical moist conditions. Both are generally referred to as 'iodized' salt.

The advantage of supplementing salt is that it is used by all sections of a community irrespective of social and economic status. It is consumed as a condiment at roughly the same level throughout the year. Its production is often confined to a few centres which means that processing can occur on a larger scale and with better controlled conditions. (Though this is often not the case in developing countries.)

The mixing of the iodine compound with salt is simple without any adverse chemical reaction. Various processes are used: dry mixing, drip feeding, and spray mixing. The dry mixing process is used in South and Central America. Drip feeding is used in India; spray mixing is becoming more widely used. All three processes use a conveyor belt. Large units producing 8–30 tons per hour of iodized salt per year need to be complemented by small units for use at village level, as in the case of the barrow method used in Vietnam.

The minimum daily requirement of iodine is only 100–150 μg per person. The level of iodization has to be sufficient to cover this requirement together with losses from the point of production to the point of consumption including the expected shelf life. It also has to take into account the per capita salt consumption in an area. There is now a view that previously generally accepted levels of salt consumption in the range 10–15 g per day are excessive because of the increased liability to hypertension. For this reason, levels in the range of 3–5 g per day are being recommended in Western countries. Iodized salt is also needed as a feed supplement for cattle and other livestock in iodine deficient areas.

Allowing for these factors, the level of iodate being used at present to provide 150 μg of iodine per day is in the range of 20–60 mg per kg. However, the concentration is likely to be further increased in the future because of concern about hypertension. A recent joint WHO/UNICEF/ICCIDD Task Force in Africa has recommended a level of 100 mg per kg in order to achieve effective control of iodine deficiency (Hetzel 1988).

The packaging of the iodized salt is very important. Jute bags have been used extensively, but in humid conditions the salt absorbs moisture. The iodate dissolves and will drip out of the bag if it is porous, resulting in a heavy loss; this has been found to reach 75 per cent over a period of nine months. To avoid this, waterproofing is required. This may be achieved by a polythene lining inside the jute bag, or else a plastic bag. The additional cost of plastic bags (50–80 per cent more) would be justified by reduced losses and their resale value.

The cost of iodization of salt is made up of the components of the chemicals, processing, packaging, and amortization of the plant. It averages at US $4.00 per ton without packaging and $8.00 per ton with packaging. The cost per 1000 population is in the range of US $20–40/year or 2–4 US cents per person per year.

Strategy for effective salt iodization

The preparation of iodized salt is only the first stage of the social process by which it eventually reaches the consumer. The likelihood of an effective salt iodization programme depends on the salt production and distribution process in the particular country. This needs to be analysed carefully prior to the initiation of a programme. It will enable the incorporation of the iodization process with the minimum disruption of the existing system of salt production and distribution. Monitoring of the iodine content at the origin, the final distribution point, and in the kitchen of the consumer, is necessary to ensure quality control. Delays in transit and exposure to heat (which will cause volatilization of iodine) and moisture, will cause variation in the concentration of iodine available for consumption. A simple method for checking the iodine content of salt is available; it is used in China and needs to be more widely used in other countries.

An effective programme requires legislative and enforcement measures in addition to quality control. However, public awareness and publicity is also necessary so that there is a demand for iodized salt. This can be avoided if the iodization of salt for human consumption is made compulsory. This is the case in China but not yet the case in India, although in 1985 legislation was passed in an effort to achieve universal salt iodization by 1992. In the meantime, there is a dual market so that it is necessary to persuade Indians living in iodine deficient areas to purchase and use iodated salt. A major media campaign has recently been mounted to achieve this in Uttar Pradesh. This features the IDD concept and the social and economic benefits to be obtained from an IDD control programme. This aspect is discussed further in the next chapter.

Present status of iodized salt programmes

Iodized salt was first introduced in Switzerland and in the USA in the 1920s when it was shown to be a successful measure (see further Chapter 1). New Zealand followed in 1941 but only very low levels were used in the first 20 years. Then in the 1950s and 60s a number of European countries followed with the expected benefits.

In general, iodization of salt was a simple procedure in these countries because the salt industries were large operations with automated refining plants. The addition of iodine was possible at very little extra cost and production could be readily achieved.

It was with confidence from this experience that salt iodization programmes were initiated in several Central and South American countries. In Guatemala, Colombia, Argentina, and Chile considerable progress was made with the control of IDD. However in

Bolivia, Ecuador, and Peru, the IDD problem has persisted. It is disturbing to note that fact that there is recent evidence of recurrence of the IDD problem in Guatemala and Colombia associated with social and political unrest. The initiation and successful maintenance of a public health programme is clearly dependent on political stability.

In the Asian countries, salt iodization has not been generally successful, even after promising pilot programmes such as the initial study in the Kangra Valley in India carried out between 1956 and 1972 (Sooch *et al.* 1973).

The Kangra Valley (Himachal Pradesh) is in the Himalayan foothills. This study area was divided into Zones A, B, and C. After a baseline survey in 1956, the salt distributed to zones A and C was fortified with potassium iodide and potassium iodate respectively, while zone B was supplied with unfortified salt. The salt fortification was such as to supply approximately 200 μg of iodine per head per day. After 6 years of iodization, i.e. in 1962, a striking decrease in the prevalence of goitre was observable in Zone A (from 38 per cent to 19 per cent) and Zone C (from 38 per cent to 15 per cent), but

Table 7.1 *Effect of iodized salt on the prevalence of goitre in schoolchildren (Kangra Valley, India)*

Zone	Sex	Prevalence of goitre (%)[a]		
		1956	*1962*	*1968*
A	male	34.1	19.3	7.5
		(2019)	(2539)	(1683)
	female	51.4	18.4	10.4
		(510)	(956)	(822)
B	male	34.2	39.8	17.2
		(1605)	(3262)	(1507)
	female	51.7	41.5	17.0
		(422)	(1282)	(1032)
C	male	36.0	14.5	8.4
		(2338)	(2527)	(1821)
		47.4	14.9	10.6
	female	(626)	(893)	(856)

[a] Figures in parentheses indicate the number examined

From Sooch *et al.* (1973), with permission.

no significant change in Zone B. Six years later in 1968, a systematic survey of goitre prevalence showed further reduction in Zone A and Zone C (8.5 per cent and 9.1 per cent respectively) (Table 7.1). In 1972, spot checks on goitre prevalence in the iodized areas by an independent group of physicians showed negligible prevalence of goitre among school children while ^{131}I uptake and urinary excretion of iodide had become normal, indicating normal thyroid function and iodine nutrition.

Following the successful Kangra Valley pilot study, the Government of India between 1962 and 1965 installed, with the financial assistance of UNICEF, a total of 12 iodization plants in different parts of the country. The concentration of iodate in salt was standardized at 25 parts per million. In 10 g of salt, the iodate supplement at this concentration amounts to 250 μg which is equivalent to 150 μg of iodine. In India, the average daily consumption of salt per head is 10 to 15 g (Pandav and Kochupillai 1982), which would give 225 μg of iodine per day. This meets the daily requirement of iodine suggested by a WHO seminar on goitre control held in 1967.

However, there have been great difficulties in the transfer of these successful results with populations of thousands to populations of millions. A review of the IDD control situation by the Nutrition Foundation of India in 1983 reveal a major short-fall in production. In fact only 15 per cent of the total requirement for iodated salt was being covered.

The failure to achieve an effective programme in India has had an adverse effect on neighbouring countries with substantial IDD problems. These include Burma, Thailand, and Bangladesh, where pilot programmes have not been followed up.

In China however, remarkable progress has been achieved since 1978 since the passing of the Cultural Revolution. Over one-third of the total population is living in an iodine deficient environment and therefore at risk of IDD. Review in 1984 indicated that at least 330 000 000 were at risk. This whole population has been supplied (mainly with iodized salt) but there is a lack of monitoring so that effective control could be demonstrated in only 6 provinces out of 27 provinces with an IDD problem (see Chapter 12).

In Africa very few programmes had been initiated prior to 1987.

These disappointing results in developing countries have to be appraised in order to plan more effectively for the future. A series of problems has become apparent as pointed out by V.K. Mannar (1987):

1. The perception of the people and the national governments of countries with a severe IDD problem has been dominated by gross ignorance of the consequences of iodine deficiency to normal growth and development.

2. In many countries salt continues to be produced along traditional semi-agricultural lines mainly by solar evaporation of sea water, lake water, or underground water in shallow ponds. Individual fields are small and worked by farmers who are not under any form of government regulation or registration.

3. The quality of salt produced is poor and is often sold in loose form without proper packaging. When the salt is iodized, transported, and stored under humid conditions most of the iodine leaches out of the salt by the time it reaches the consumer.

4. Erratic and unknown distribution patterns also make it difficult to monitor the movement of salt. The iodized salt is more expensive than the uniodized salt so that the poorer people who are more vulnerable to IDD are more likely to prefer the latter.

5. At government level there is inadequate programme management. Legislation has often been ineffective due to failure of enforcement.

These failures had become apparent by the mid 1970s but there was continued inaction at government level. The new awareness of the extent of the IDD problem in the 1980s has led to a serious reappraisal, and recent significant initiatives have been taken in a number of Asian countries (see Chapter 12). However, the difficulties in salt iodination already listed will not easily or quickly be overcome. This applies particularly to 2; 3; and 4.

An example is the island of Java in Indonesia with a population of 100 million. There, only 30 per cent of the salt production is under government control. The other 70 per cent is controlled by a myriad of small producers marketing, in general, poor quality salt. Iodization of the salt produced by these small producers is not feasible. An alternative is required. This leads us to the other modalities of iodine supplementation.

Iodized oil

The history of injections of iodized oil has been described in Chapter 4. Since the initial work in New Guinea, iodized oil injections have been used on a vast scale, particularly in Indonesia, China, Burma, Nepal (Fig. 7.1) and Zaire. More recently, extensive campaigns have been conducted in Bolivia, Peru, and Pakistan (Dunn 1987).

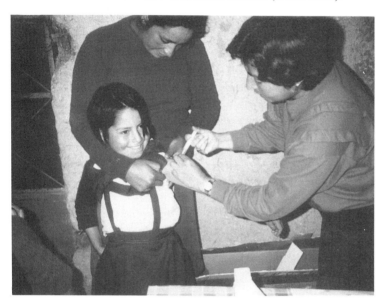

Fig. 7.1. Young girl receiving an injection of iodized oil in Nepal—she is quite relaxed about it! (By courtesy of Dr John T. Dunn, with permission.)

The peculiar advantage of iodized oil is its applicability to remote or isolated situations such as mountain areas—as in the original situation in Papua New Guinea. Such situations pose obstructions to the distribution of any food items, including salt. There is usually a subsistence economy with the consumption of locally grown food-stuffs from iodine deficient soils (Buttfield and Hetzel 1967).

In Papua New Guinea, the iodized oil injections were given by mobile patrols moving through the villages or by the Aid Post

Orderly (APO), who was the 'backbone' of the public health service. He was usually responsible for the basic health care of about 1000 people living in an average of 7 villages (see Chapter 4).

In Indonesia, the injections were given mainly by specially trained health workers who also carried out goitre surveys and have been responsible for extensive data collections for the evaluation of the programme. In addition the primary health care village workers have been involved. But the programme could not have been carried out without specifically trained health workers.

In China, most of the injections were given by 'barefoot doctors' who provided a large source of readily available manpower. Barefoot doctors are part-time health workers who have been selected by their local village communities (in China 80 per cent of the population lives in rural areas) for short courses of training of 1–2 months and then return to their villages to provide basic health care. They have been the main providers of health care at village level in China for the past 30 years.

In Zaire, there were no basic health services in the iodine deficient areas, so mobile teams were used. Each team of five persons gave about 500 injections per day making a total of 100 000 per year. This permitted the coverage of 1.5 million people in five years. Overall direction came from a coordinating epidemiologist.

Chemistry and pharmacology

Iodized oil can be prepared because iodine can be attached chemically to the double bond between carbon atoms of unsaturated fatty acids which are found most commonly in vegetable oils. The chemical reaction is a simple one and easily carried out. Any one of a variety of vegetable oils can be used. The most widely available commercial preparation is Lipiodol (made by Laboratoire Guerbet in Paris), which is a poppyseed oil with 38 per cent of its weight as iodine; 1 ml of this product contains 480 mg iodine. This oil is distributed in the USA as Ethiodol and in Europe as Neohyriol, but all the production is undertaken by Guerbet.

The only other major source is China where the Fourth Pharmaceutical Company of Wuhan has produced a preparation which contains 24–28 per cent, iodine and capsules for oral use containing 200 mg iodine each.

The oil is given by intramuscular injection (usually in the upper arm). Absorption into the blood occurs slowly so that most of it remains at the site for weeks or months. One study using Lipiodol labelled with radio-iodine showed that 87 per cent of the iodine was still at the site of injection 23 days later. Once in the blood stream the iodine can be taken up by the thyroid, excreted in the urine, and stored in the fatty tissue of the body (Buttfield and Hetzel 1967; Dunn 1987).

If the oil is given by mouth, it is absorbed directly into the blood stream as iodized oil. Some is deiodized in the liver and other tissues and the iodine is taken up by the thyroid or excreted by the kidney. The rest is incorporated into fatty tissue as normally occurs with the fatty acids from the foods. The iodine stored in the fat is then slowly released over several months.

In Papua New Guinea doses of 4 ml (nearly 2 g iodine) were used without ill effect in a population of the order of about 120 000. The results of the initial studies are shown in Figs. 4.8 and Table 7.2. It will be seen that a single iodized oil injection was able to restore to normal the low level of PBI (the measure of thyroxine in the blood) for a period of up to four and a half years. A further advantage was the disappearance of goitre within 1–3 months as already noted (Fig. 4.9). This caused considerable satisfaction to the local community when first observed by them and led to enthusiastic acceptance of the oil (Buttfield and Hetzel 1967).

Table 7.2 *The effect of iodized oil on thyroid function in New Guinea subjects*†

Group	Urinary iodine ($\mu g/24$ h)	^{131}I uptake (% at 24 h)	Serum PBI ($\mu g/100$ ml)
Untreated	11.5 ± 12.4 (91)	70 ± 19 (181)	4.1 ± 2.1 (204)
Treated 18 months before	119 ± 114 (18)	31 ± 20 (51)	8.2 ± 2.6 (27)
Treated 3 years before	35 ± 25 (29)	37 ± 19 (43)	7.8 ± 1.6 (52)
Treated 4½ years before	23 ± 21 (11)	44 ± 18 (67)	6.4 ± 2.4 (43)
Australian normal range	70–140	16–40	3.6–7.2

Modified from Buttfield and Hetzel (1967), with permission.
† Statistical analysis showed highly significant differences between the treated and untreated groups in urinary iodine. ^{131}I uptake, and serum PBI (P < 0.001).

As the populations covered have increased, the dosage has been reduced to lower levels. Recent recommendations are 0.5 ml for children in the first year of life and 1 ml for all older subjects. Several studies from Latin America and Africa have shown that 1 ml will correct iodine deficiency for a minimum of 3 years. A dose of 3 ml will give coverage for 3–4 years. A larger dose will be indicated if the iodine deficient community lives in a more remote area because of the transport costs of the mobile injection team.

In all, in excess of 12 million injections of iodized oil have been given in the last 15 years with very little in the way of side effects apart from a rare abscess at the site of injection. 'Cold chain' (refrigerator) is not required, which is a great advantage. Iodized oil is certainly an effective means for the correction of iodine deficiency and has opened up the possibility of elimination of IDD as a public health problem in the next decade.

However, the necessity for an injection has been questioned, in view of the costs of the syringe and needles and the necessity to have specially trained staff to give the injections. If the staff are readily available through the primary health care system, then the costs are comparable to those of iodated salt: 5–10 US cents per person per year. On the other hand, if the oil could be given orally it would be possible to use village health volunteers to supervise the administration. This would make it much more available to village communities with severe IDD problems. Another advantage of the oral preparation is the freedom from the risk of AIDS or hepatitis B infection from contaminated syringes, although this should be eliminated by proper sterilization of needles or by using disposable syringes. Recent seminars such as the 1987 Joint WHO/UNICEF/ICCIDD Regional Seminar in Africa have pointed out the convenience of oral administration at yearly intervals through the primary health care system at village level (Hetzel 1987).

There is less experience with oral iodized oil than with the injection. However, there are now ten studies of its use with 200–960 mg for a single dose. Coverage was 1–2 years for a dose of 1–2 ml, approximately half the period that would be covered by the intramuscular injection.

One question that arises with the oral oil is whether it would be adequately absorbed in the presence of coincident intestinal disease with malabsorption. This needs to be further investigated. Low fat stores in the body would also reduce the period of coverage.

The position at this time is that the oral administration of iodized oil has been shown to be effective in the correction of severe iodine deficiency—a dose of 1 ml (480 mg iodine) would provide cover for one year, and 2 ml for three years. In less severe endemics with urinary iodine levels of 50 μg per day, 1 ml for two years would be satisfactory.

So far the only sources of production of iodized oil are the two already mentioned, Laboratoire Guerbet of Paris and the Fourth Pharmaceutical Company of Wuhan in China. Another source is urgently required. Efforts to produce the oil have now begun in several countries (India, Indonesia, and Australia), so it is hoped that a suitable preparation will soon available. What is required is an industrial process at minimum cost so that oil can be available for mass use as a nutrition supplement. A number of vegetable oils would be suitable vehicles and a selection could be made of the cheapest and most readily available form for the particular country undertaking production. It is also clear that economies of scale could be secured by one country producing oil for neighbouring countries as well as for itself. Recent developments involving collaboration between Indonesia and Australia towards the production of an iodized peanut oil are described in Chapter 12.

Target groups

An iodized oil supplementation programme is necessary when other methods have been found ineffective or can be considered to be inapplicable. Iodized oil can be regarded as an emergency measure until an effective iodized salt programme can be introduced. The spectacular and rapid effects of iodized oil in reducing goitre can be important in demonstrating the benefits of iodization, which can lead to community demand for iodized salt.

In the light of the evidence from Papua New Guinea, Zaire and national IDD control programmes, the major groups requiring iodized oil are:

1. women of reproductive age;
2. children between 0 and 5 years of age;
3. children up to completion of adolescence (16 years).

In general, iodized oil should be avoided over the age of 45 because of the possibility of precipitating hyperthyroidism as discussed later in this chapter. Pregnancy is not regarded as a contra-indication.

It is desirable for the male population to be included in an iodized oil programme even though the other groups already mentioned are more at risk. Males include the leaders in village communities. Their experience of the benefits will include greater productivity and quality of life which are important to community acceptance.

Cost

There is a considerable variation in the costs in various parts of the world, as might be expected. One important factor is the availability of primary health care staff for the administration of the oil whether by mouth or injection. If existing staff are available then the cost of iodized oil injections is comparable to that of iodized salt.

In 1983, Lipiodol cost 13 French francs (US $1.60) per 10 ml or 0.16 US cents per dose of 1 ml which would be adequate cover for 2–3 years by injection (or 8 US cents per year) which compares with 2–4 US cents per year for iodized salt. In 1985, the cost of oil in Bolivia was US $2.38 for a 10 ml phial. In Indonesia in 1983 the iodized oil injection programme cost US $1.00 per injection (3 ml) including administration costs. Iodized oil could be prepared more cheaply for oral use.

An important feature of iodized oil administration is that it can be carried out without the legislation required for iodized salt.

The possibility of linking up an iodized oil programme with other preventive programmes including the Child Immunization Programme, is now under active consideration. Great progress has been made with child immunization programmes in Africa and Asia. A series of injections are given covering triple antigen (diphtheria, tetanus toxoid, and whooping cough) (3 injections), polio (usually double oral administration), and measles (single injection). The target group is young children (0–2 years). Tetanus toxoid is recommended for pregnant women as a preventive measure against tetanus in the neonate.

To this series of measures iodized oil could readily be added to cover young children over the first 2–5 years of life—the second most important target group. Women would require separate coverage, possibly through the family planning health care system.

Iodized bread

Iodized bread has been used in Holland and in Australia. Detailed observations are available from Tasmania (Clements *et al.* 1970).

Since 1949 the Tasmanian population has received a number of intended and unintended iodine dietary supplements. These began in 1949 with the use of weekly tablets of potassium iodide (10 mg) given to infants, children, and pregnant women through baby health clinics, schools, and antenatal clinics whenever possible.

The prevalence of endemic goitre fell progressively over these 16 years but was not eliminated. This was traced to lack of cooperation by a number of schools in the distribution of the iodide tablets. The distribution through the child health centres to infants and pre-school children was also ineffective because of their irregular attendance.

For this reason a decision was made to change the method of prophylaxis from iodide tablets to iodization of bread. The use of potassium iodate up to 20 parts per million (ppm) as a bread improver was authorized by the National Health and Medical Research Council of Australia in 1963, and the necessary legislation was passed by the Tasmanian Parliament in 1964.

The effect of bread iodization was followed by a series of surveys of palpable goitre in schoolchildren. A definite effect on visible goitre rate was apparent by 1969. Studies of urinary iodide excretion and plasma inorganic iodide in May 1967, revealed no excessive intake of iodide. Correction of iodine deficiency was confirmed by evidence of a fall in 24-hour radio-iodine uptake levels in hospital subjects, as well as by normal plasma inorganic iodine concentration and urine iodine excretion (Stewart *et al.* 1971).

It may be concluded that bread iodization was effective in correcting iodine deficiency in Tasmania in the 1960s. However, there is now a much greater diversity of sources for dietary iodine. Iodine is readily available from milk due to the use of iodophors in the dairy industry. It is also available from ice-cream due to the use of alginate as a thickener. These factors mean that the risk of iodine deficiency has diminished greatly in the West.

Water iodization

Reduction in goitre rate from 61 per cent to 30 per cent with 79 per cent of goitres showing visible reduction has been demonstrated following iodization of the water supply in Sarawak. Significant rises in serum T_4 and falls in TSH were also shown. Urinary iodine excretions indicated iodine repletion (Maberly *et al.* 1981).

Similar results have been obtained with preliminary studies in

Thailand by Dr Romsai Suwanik and his group at the Siriraj Hospital, Bangkok (1983) and Squatrito *et al* (1986) in Sicily.

It is suggested that iodized water may be more convenient than iodized salt and there is the additional benefit of the antiseptic action. This method is appropriate at village level if a specific source of drinking water can be identified, otherwise there is a heavy cost, as less than 1 per cent of a general water supply is used for drinking purposes.

Other methods

In Bangkok, Dr Romsai Suwanik has also developed iodized fish sauce and iodized soya sauce. These sauces are also being used for iron supplementation.

In the original controlled trial in Ohio schoolchildren (1917–1922), Marine and Kimball used 200 mg sodium iodide in water daily for 10 days in the spring and repeated this in the autumn. Satisfactory regression of goitre was observed. In Tasmania, Clements *et al.* (1968) used 10 mg of potassium iodide tablets weekly through schools and child health centres with some (but an irregular) regression of goitre. Failure of reduction of goitre was attributed to inadequate cooperation in the schools and health centres and led to the introduction of bread iodization in 1966.

The intermittent use of oral iodide tablets certainly should be considered as an option in schoolchildren for moderate iodine deficiency, where compliance can be more readily enforced than in adults. However, oral iodized oil offers a more reliable alternative because it would be administered only once in one or two years depending on the dosage.

The hazards of iodization

A mild increase in incidence of (hyperthyroidism thyrotoxicosis) has been described following iodized salt programmes in Europe and South America and following the introduction of iodized bread in Holland and Tasmania. A few cases have been noted following iodized oil administration in South America. No cases have yet been described in New Guinea, India, or Zaire. This is probably due to the scattered nature of the population in small villages and limited opportunities for observation. The condition is largely confined to those over 40 years of age (Connolly *et al.* 1970). It is due to elevated levels of thyroid hormones which produce a rapid heart rate and other features of a nervous state (trembling, excessive sweating, instability and less of weight).

In Tasmania it was apparent that the rise in incidence of thyrotoxicosis had occurred in association with a rise in iodine intake from below normal to normal levels due to iodized bread which was introduced in April 1966. The group affected was composed mainly of those over the age of 40 with life-long iodine deficiency causing autonomous thyroid glands to continue the rapid turnover of iodine after the increase in iodine intake. The condition can be readily controlled with antithyroid drugs or radio-iodine. It seems likely that spontaneous remission occurs in many cases. In general iodization should be minimized for those over the age of 40 because of the risk of thyrotoxicosis. With control of iodine deficiency the condition disappears and hence it is classified as an iodine deficiency disorder.

General comment

The methods available for iodine supplementation fall into two categories:

1. measures for the whole population—iodized salt, bread, and water;
2. prescriptive measures suitable for children and women of reproductive age—iodized oil and iodide tablets.

The great advantage of the prescriptive approach is that it can be carried out through the health care system. It does not, as in the case of population measures, require cooperation and enforcement measures involving other government departments and private industry. For this reason, prescriptive measures (mainly iodized oil) have to be given more serious consideration than in the past when the tendency was to think iodized salt was the first choice. The importance of *quantitative* correction of severe iodine deficiency, particularly in women and children, in order to prevent 'cretinoids' requires a much more critical approach than in the past, particularly to severe iodine deficiency.

Oral administration of iodized oil to children could be carried out through the baby health centres and schools. Periods of 1–2 years could be covered at present (2 ml dose), but this period may well be increased in the light of further research. The injection will last longer (2 ml for 3–4 years) and is readily organized when it can be carried out by existing health care staff. Cheaper production of iodized oil is readily achievable and should be provided in India, Indonesia, and other countries with large populations at risk. The advantages of a single administration of iodized oil against multiple administrations of iodide tablets are obvious.

In China an iodized oil injection has been introduced for iodine deficient young women just before marriage. This will cover them for three years which would confer protection for the single pregnancy that is now in force as family planning policy in China.

The complication of iodine induced thyrotoxicosis is unavoidable for population measures. As it is more likely to occur over the age of 40, its incidence mainly depends on the proportion of the population over the age of 40 years which is a lower proportion in a developing country than in developed countries.

Summary

The advantages and disadvantages of prescription versus population measures have to be considered in every different region and within any national programme. In the massive iodine deficient populations in Asia, the great advantages of salt iodization as a population measure in the prevention of large scale mental deficiency outweigh the disadvantages of iodine induced thyrotoxicosis. However, the use of iodized oil by mouth or by injection offers a more immediate and more effective alternative for severe iodine deficiency and is recommended until iodized salt can be made effective in correcting iodine deficiency. The combination of the two measures is sufficient to ensure effective correction of iodine deficiency.

Bibliography

Buttfield, I. H. and Hetzel, B. S. (1967). Endemic goitre in Eastern New Guinea with special reference to the use of iodised oil in prophylaxis and treatment. *Bull. World Health Organization* **36**, 243–62.

Clements, F. W., Gibson, H. B., and Howeler-Coy, J. F. (1968). Goitre studies in Tasmania: 16 years prophylaxis with iodide. *Bull. World Health Organization* **38**, 297–318.

Clements, F.W., Gibson, H.B., and Howeler-Coy, J.F. (1970). Goitre prophylaxis by addition of potassium iodate to bread. Experience in Tasmania. *Lancet* 1, 489–92.

Connolly, R.J., Vidor, G.I., and Stewart, J.C. (1970). Increase in thyrotoxicosis in endemic area after iodation of bread. *Lancet* 1, 500–2.

Dunn, J.T. (1987). Iodised oil in the treatment and prophylaxis of IDD. In *The prevention and control of iodine deficiency disorders* (eds. B.S. Hetzel, J.T. Dunn, and J.B. Stanbury) pp. 127–136. Elsevier, Amsterdam.

Hetzel, B.S. (1988). Iodine deficiency disorders. *Lancet* 1, 1386–7.

Maberly, G.F., Eastman, C.J. and Corcoran, J.M. (1981). Effect of iodination of a village water-supply on goitre size and thyroid function. *Lancet* 2, 1270–2.

Mannar, V.M.G. (1987). Control of iodine deficiency disorders by iodination of salt: strategy for developing countries. In *The prevention and control of iodine deficiency disorders* (eds. B.S. Hetzel, J.T., Dunn, and J.B. Stanbury) pp. 111–126. Elsevier, Amsterdam.

Nutrition Foundation of India (1983). *The national goitre control program: a blueprint for its intensification*. Scientific Report 1, 57.

Pandav, C.S. and Kochupillai, N. (1982). Endemic goitre in India: prevalence, etiology, attendant disability and control measures. *Indian Journal of Pediatrics* 50, 259–71.

Sooch, S.S., Deo, M.G., Karmarkar, M.G., Kochupillai, N., Ramachandran, K., and Ramalingaswami, V. (1973). Prevention of endemic goitre with iodised salt. *Bull. World Health Organization* 49, 307–12.

Squatrito, S., Vigneri, R., Runello, F., Ermans, A.M., Polley, R.D., and Ingbar, S.H. (1986). Prevention and treatment of endemic iodine-deficiency goitre by iodination of a municipal water supply. *Journal of Clinical Endocrinology and Metabolism* 63, 368–74.

Stewart, J.C., Vidor, G.I., Buttfield, I.H., and Hetzel, B.S. (1971). Epidemic thyrotoxicosis in Northern Tasmania: Studies of clinical features and iodine nutrition. *Australian and New Zealand Journal of Medicine* 3, 203–11.

Suwanik, R. (1983). Personal communication, Bangkok.

WHO/UNICEF/ICCIDD 1987 Regional Seminar *Control of iodine deficiency disorders in Africa*. AFRO/WHO Regional office for Africa, Brazzaville.

Further reading

Dunn, J.T., Pretell, E.A., Daza, C.H., and Viteri, F.E. (eds.) (1986). *Towards the eradication of endemic goiter, cretinism, and iodine deficiency.* Scientific Publication No. 502. PAHO, Washington.

Hetzel, B.S., Dunn, J.T., and Stanbury, J.B. (eds.) (1987). *The prevention and control of iodine deficiency disorders.* Elsevier, Amsterdam.

Stanbury, J.B. and Hetzel, B.S. (eds.) (1980). *Endemic goiter and cretinism: iodine nutrition in health and disease.* Wiley, New York.

8

National IDD control programmes

National IDD Control Programmes are the basic functional units for the prevention and control of IDD. Global control depends on effective national control. In view of the effectiveness of the various methods for correction of iodine deficiency described in the previous chapter, it would be anticipated that national programmes would be successful.

The fact is, however, that until very recently this has not been so. In Latin America there has been some success in Guatemala and Colombia, but there is now a reversal in these countries associated with political and social unrest. In India there has been a disastrous failure in the iodation of salt such that less than a quarter of the required amount was available for human consumption in 1984. In Africa very few progammes have even been initiated until the last 2 years. Even in Europe there are persistent IDD problems of national significance in East and West Germany and Italy, as well as localized problems in many other countries. Some countries such as Indonesia and China have made significant progress.

The reasons for these frequent failures and the less frequent successes are obviously important to determine. It is clear that success in IDD control depends on much more than effective technology. It depends on an effective delivery or public health programme, which is a complex undertaking with a number of major elements. In this chapter we shall review these elements. In the subsequent chapters in Part III we shall consider national control programmes in different countries by global region. To assist description and analysis, a social process model has been developed (Fig. 8.1).

This model will now be described in detail:

(1) assessment (collecting data, assessing a situation);
(2) communication (disseminating findings);
(3) planning (developing or updating a plan of action);

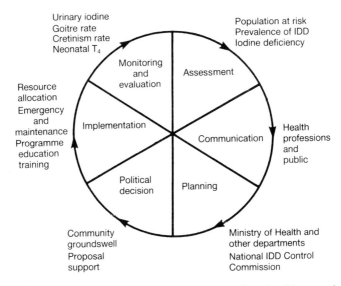

Fig. 8.1. A model showing the social process involved in a national IDD control programme. Success depends on the establishment of a national IDD control commission with full political and legislative authority to carry it out. (From Hetzel 1987, with permission.)

(4) political decision (achieving political will and obtaining support);
(5) implementation;
(6) monitoring and evaluation.

The process then begins a further cycle with new data, dissemination of the results of the first programme, and development of a modified new one to correct the deficiencies of the first (Hetzel 1987).

Assessment

In public health programmes carrying out iodine supplementation, the first problem is to assess a population or group living in an area that is suspected of being iodine deficient. The data required include the following:

(1) the total population, including the number of children under 15 years of age (when the effects of IDD are so important);
(2) the goitre rate, including the rates of palpable or visible goitre;
(3) the rates of cretinism and 'cretinoidism' in the population;
(4) the level of urinary iodine excretion;
(5) the level of iodine in the drinking water;
(6) the level of serum thyroxine (T_4) in various age groups. Particular attention is now focused on the levels in the neonate because of the importance of the T_4 level for early brain development.

Basic population data are usually available and make a reference point of obvious importance in developing an iodization programme if it is to be comprehensive. There are difficulties in reaching the whole iodine deficient population, especially because of the remoteness of many communities. Observing schoolchildren has obvious advantages of access and convenience and has been extensively reported (Fig. 8.2).

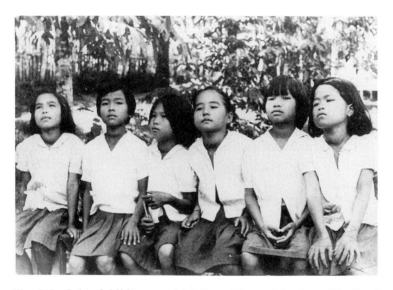

Fig. 8.2. Schoolchildren aged 10 from Phrae, Northern Thailand with goitre. (Courtesy of Dr R. Suwanik, Bangkok.)

A classification of goitre severity has been adopted by the World Health Organization. There are still minor differences in technique among different observers. In general, visible goitre is more readily verified than the palpable type. The most recent authoritative review of the classification of goitre and cretinism was carried out at the PAHO/WHO meeting in Lima, November 1983, and was published by WHO (Dunn *et al.* 1986). The following extract is taken from that review:

Definition of goitre stages

A. Definition of goitre

A normal thyroid gland should have the minimal size compatible with euthyroidism under conditions of normal iodine intake (100–150 mg/day). This gland would be non-palpable or barely palpable. For practical purposes, the definition of goitre of Perez *et al.* (1960) is recommended: 'A thyroid gland whose lateral lobes have a volume greater than the terminal phalanges of the thumbs of the person examined will be considered goitrous.

B. Estimation of thyroid size

A slight modification of the system of Perez *et al.* (1960) is recommended:

Stage 0	No goitre.
Stage 1a	Goitre detectable.
Stage 1b	Goitre palpable and visible only when the neck is fully extended. This stage also includes nodular glands, even if not goitrous; see Section C below.
Stage 2	Goitre visible with the neck in normal position; palpation is not needed for diagnosis.
Stage 3	Very large goitre that can be recognized at a considerable distance.

In case of doubt between any two of these stages, the lower should be recorded.

Measurement of thyroid surfaces by the procedure of MacLennan and Gaitan (1974) is particularly recommended for standardization of technique among different examiners and for comparison of surveys in different areas at different times.

The total goitre rate is the prevalence of stages 1–3; the visible goitre rate is the prevalence of stages 2–3. This classification is appropriate to field surveys for public health purposes. For clinical purposes, more precise information can be obtained by other techniques including scintigraphy and sonography.

C. Estimation of the consistency of the thyroid by palpation
The diffuse or nodular consistency of the thyroid should be recorded. Nodules usually occur in areas where marked iodine deficiency has been long-standing. This estimation should be independent of that for the size of the thyroid, with the following exception: when one or more nodules are found in a non-goitrous gland, it will be recorded as Stage 1b since nodularity implies marked modifications in the structure of the gland.

Definition of IDD as a public health problem

An area is arbitrarily defined as endemic with respect to goitre if more than 10 per cent of the population or of the children aged six to twelve years are found to be goitrous. The figure 10 per cent was chosen because a higher prevalence usually implies an environmental factor, while a prevalence of several per cent is common even when all known environment factors are controlled.

Endemic cretinism and additional developmental abnormalities

A. Definition by three main features

1. *Epidemiology*. It is associated with endemic goitre and severe iodine deficiency.
2. *Clinical manifestations*. These comprise mental deficiency together with either:

    a. a predominant neurological syndrome including defects of hearing and speech, squint, and characteristic disorders of stance and gait of varying degree;

    or,

    b. predominant hypothyroidism and stunted growth.

    Although in some regions one of the two types may predominate, in other areas a combination of the two syndromes will occur.
3. *Prevention*. In areas where adequate correction of iodine deficiency has been achieved, endemic cretinism has been prevented.

B. Other developmental abnormalities

It has now become increasingly clear that endemic cretinism represents only the extreme stage of a broader spectrum of developmental abnormalities including decreased intellectual potential.

These abnormalities are also prevented by correction of iodine deficiency (see Chapter 6).

The rates of cretinoids and 'cretinoidism' may be difficult to determine. Observations of schoolchildren will not detect those most severely affected who are likely not to be attending school. Studies of IQ provide additional important evidence justifying programmes.

Urinary iodine excretion can be determined appropriately on 24-hour samples. The difficulties of collection may be insurmountable, however. For this reason, as originally suggested by Follis (1964), determinations are made on casual samples from a group of approximately 30 subjects. The iodine levels are expressed as $\mu g/g$ of creatinine excretion and the range plotted out as a histogram. This provides a reference point for the level of iodine excretion which is also a good index of the level of iodine nutrition. Modern automated equipment (autoanalyser) is making the analysis of large numbers of samples quite feasible. Methods have been recently improved so that reliable results can be obtained.

It has been suggested that there are three grades of severity of IDD in a population that may be determined by urinary iodine excretion (Hetzel 1987). These are as follows:

Mild IDD   Goitre endemias with an average of iodine excretion of more than $50 \mu g/g$ of creatinine. At this level, a thyroid hormone supply adequate for normal mental and physical development can be anticipated. Iodized salt is the appropriate correction measure. Economic development alone might also achieve this.

Moderate IDD   Goitre endemias with an average urinary iodine excretion of between 25 and $50 \mu g/g$ of creatinine. In these circumstances, adequate thyroid hormone formation may be impaired. This group is at risk of hypothyroidism but not of overt cretinism; iodized salt may be adequate but if effective salt iodization cannot be achieved quickly, iodized oil is indicated.

Severe IDD   Goitre endemias with an average urinary iodine excretion below $25 \mu g/g$ of creatinine. Endemic cretinism is a serious risk in such a population.

Iodized oil is required for quantitative correction
and will need to be continued if subsistence agriculture continues in the area.

The level of iodine in drinking water indicates the level of iodine
in the soil, which in turn determines the level of iodine in the crops
and animals in the area. Water iodine levels in deficient areas are
usually below 2 μg/l.

The level of serum thyroxine (T_4) provides an indirect measure of
iodine nutritional status. Radio-immunoassay methods with automated equipment have greatly assisted this approach. Particular
attention should be given to levels of blood T_4 in the neonate;
levels below 4 μg per cent must be regarded as prejudicial to brain
development.

Communication

Communication is concerned with transmitting the message of the
effects of iodine deficiency to various target groups that make up a
community. There are three major categories to be considered.

(1) *Health professionals*: both within and outside the public sector;
(2) *Politicians*: Policy and decision makers;
(3) *General public*: in many countries includes diverse groups with
    different cultural backgrounds.

Health professionals

Health professionals have been educated in an earlier time when the
concept of the effects of iodine deficiency was simply 'goitre'. The
broader IDD concept has so far had only limited circulation within
the large health professional group. The fact is that IDD covers a
wide diversity of effects that overlaps a number of special health and
health service areas. These include maternal and child health,
mental health, family planning, and nutrition. The IDD message
needs to reach health professionals in all these fields and the prevention and control of IDD to be incorporated into their programmes.

Suitable textual material is now becoming available. The first
ICCIDD monograph on '*The prevention and control of iodine deficiency disorders* was specifically designed for the multidisciplinary
audience that health professionals now comprise. These include
administrators, planners, economists, and statisticians, as well as

medical graduates in public health and epidemiology. Then there are the nutritionists, nurses, and technicians in laboratories and clinics who also need to have an understanding of IDD.

Finally, there is a special category who are not health professionals; these include the salt technologists and administrators in the salt industry. It is of interest that the European group of salt manufacturers has recently decided to establish a 'Salt and Health Committee' with representatives from a number of European countries from both health and salt industry sectors.

Politicans, policy and decision makers

This group is exceedingly important because it controls the allocation of funds for public health programmes and decides on the relative merits of different areas in a limited national, state, or regional budget.

It is important to recognize that this group has no interest in the detailed physiological effects of iodine deficiency through reduction of thyroid hormone output. These matters are for health professionals. The interest of policy and decision makers is in the operational benefits of iodine deficiency control. What does prevention of IDD mean in terms of improved perinatal mortality, improved school performance, improved health and well-being of the adults both male and female which might be reflected in increased work output and productivity as well as an improved quality of life? Such questions are very important for Third World countries as Nepal because of the rigours of life in the hills and mountains of the Himalayas. Cretins are handicapped people who are unable to 'pull their weight'. In this and other iodine deficient regions they are unable to feed themselves so they have to be looked after by others, which represents a significant burden on the family and local community (Levin 1987).

The general apathy of severely iodine deficient communities and its removal by correction of the deficiency is clearly very important in the political arena. Correction of iodine deficiency will lead to greater self-reliance and individual and social initiative, as we have seen in the Chinese village of Jixian.

The use of modern methods of communication such as films and videos is now increasing in the health area, and IDD has been the subject of several films made by the UNICEF office in Delhi (regional office for South and Central Asia). The most recent film on IDD in Asia includes footage from Bhutan, Nepal, India, Indonesia, and China. It is designed for policy and decision makers. It has a powerful impact with the emphasis on the feasibility of prevention of the severe disabilities of cretinism. Such a video should be shown on national television networks to arouse awareness of the IDD message both in the Third World and in the developed world.

It is the author's hope that this book on *The story of iodine deficiency* will also increase awareness of the IDD problem in a wide audience beyond the health professional group.

General public

We have to distinguish between an educated public able to read, that is more likely urban, and an uneducated group who cannot read and is more likely to be rural. It is the latter group that is likely to have IDD. For such groups the transistor radio and television are very important aids to communication.

In the case of the general community it is obvious that the IDD message has to be presented in pragmatic, down to earth terms, as to what prevention and control means in terms of child survival, child development, school performance, productivity, and quality of life. Just as for the politicians, the technique for communication will vary depending on the educational status of the group.

Recent experience with public health programmes indicates the importance of studying community perceptions of particular problems, and then designing on approach which takes into account these community perceptions. The term 'social marketing' refers to this approach which has now become a prominent feature of public health programmes, particularly in the Third World.

One of the foremost exponents of social marketing is Richard K. Manoff of Manoff International Inc., New York. Manoff (1987) points out that the usual presentation using the problem–solution approach may be inappropriate for the target audience. The perception of the target audience of the problem might be quite different to that of the health professional. As an interesting example, Manoff cites the promotion of iodized salt over the radio in Ecuador in 1973. The following recorded dialogue was broadcast by local radio in Quechua—

MUSIC:	*THEME IN UP AND UNDER*
ANNOUNCER:	Better mothers raise better children. A story about a little thing like salt.
MUSIC:	*UP AND UNDER*
MOTHER:	Doctor, why is my new baby not normal?
DOCTOR:	Because of your coto.
MOTHER:	Coto is nothing. Many people in my village have coto.
DOCTOR:	Coto is a sickness. In a woman, coto can damage her unborn child. It is caused by not enough iodine in your food.
MOTHER:	What is iodine?
DOCTOR:	A secret element of foods like fish and iodized salt. Every one must have iodine to be healthy—to prevent coto.
MOTHER:	We eat fish sometimes. And I use salt *all* the time.
DOCTOR:	Not just salt. *Iodized* salt.
MOTHER:	Yes—the sal en grano.
DOCTOR:	No. Sal yodado. The white salt in the plastic package.
MOTHER:	Ah. . . . (sadly) Salt. . . . such a little thing. Sal yadado. . . . such an important thing.
MUSIC:	*UP AND OUT*
ANNOUNCER:	You can prevent coto. Always use sal yodado, the white salt in the plastic package for the whole family. It costs a little more. But it does so much more.

This message was broadcast several times a day for most of the year. The first exchange between mother and doctor aims to change the popular perception of 'coto' (Quechua for 'goitre') as a normal condition to an awareness of its significance for the unborn child during pregnancy. In effect, as Manoff points out, IDD had to be discovered by the audience! The perception of goitre as normal because indeed it affected some 30 per cent of the local population, would clearly be a 'resistance point' to the use of iodized salt when it became available. So the promotion effort had to take this into account if iodized salt was to be successfully introduced.

The second phase of the dialogue is concerned with iodine. 'What is iodine?' the mother asks and then with the explanation, iodized salt ('Sal yodado') is mentioned and the difference between non-iodized salt and iodized salt is explained. Finally there is a promotion of 'Sal yodado' by the announcer after the earlier messages have been communicated.

Such considerations are not irrelevant to communication with politicians who have to be closer to public perception than health professionals usually are! Manoff points out that presentations to politicians and decision-makers can easily suffer from overkill with too much data including 'dry as dust' facts and statistics. This is relevant to presentation of cases for IDD in the competition for allocation of resources in the public health sector.

Currently, a major media programme is underway in Uttar Pradesh, to persuade the community to used iodated salt. The consumer is being taken seriously for the first time in India. (By contrast in China, most of the salt is iodized and no media campaign is necessary in that society where there is in general a much more limited range of choices.) In Uttar Pradesh, the television coverage is limited. This means that mobile audiovisual aids are the most appropriate media for dissemination and communication. However, all possible techniques will have to be mobilized. Posters, cinema, radio, and press are all being used. Approaches through song and drama are also being developed. Mobile vans with videos have been organized. Uttar Pradesh has a total population of 110 million of which at least 50 per cent are at risk of IDD due to living in a seriously iodine deficient area. So there is a considerable challenge!

Successful pilot projects are being recognized as a means to mobilize community support. In Bangladesh a pilot iodized oil injection programme in 1977 and again in 1983 caused visible reduction of goitre and the birth of normal children to mothers who had previously had miscarriages and produced subnormal babies. As a result, many village populations who had been suspicious and fearful of injections are now keen to have them.

An example of village education material from Pakistan is shown in Fig. 8.3.

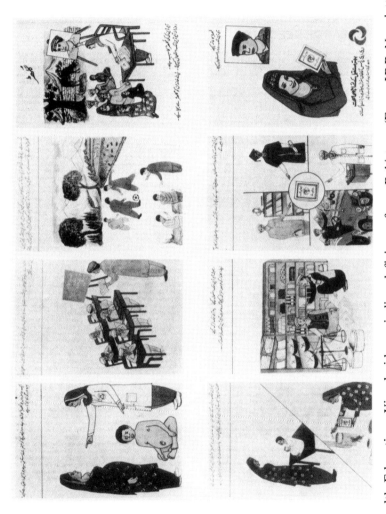

Fig. 8.3 Health Education: Visual aids on iodine deficiency from Pakistan. (From *IDD Newsletter*, Vol. 3, No. 2, 1987, and Aga Khan Foundation, with permission.)

Planning

Planning an IDD control programme is clearly of concern to a country's department of health. It is now recognized that most public health programmes require an 'intersectoral' approach which involves a number of government departments. These include education and communication, as we have seen from the previous section; industry and commerce (in relation to salt production and distribution); and the agricultural section because of the importance of iodine deficiency for livestock. In addition, a number of different sections of the health department, nutrition, maternal and child health, and mental health, should be involved. There also needs to be consultation with the community at large to increase awareness of the community perceptions relevant to the IDD problem.

All these considerations are best met if a national IDD control commission is appointed by the government through the minister of health. This commission should have political authority to carry out the programme. Its Chairman should be nominated by the government with delegation of this authority. The membership can then reflect the various government departments and the private sector. University representation is also useful to provide an academic and research input. The responsibility of the national commission is essentially to develop the IDD control programme as laid out in the social process cycle (Fig. 8.1).

The planning needs to specify objectives for the correction of iodine deficiency; alternative or multiple strategies for achieving objectives; and priorities in the light of the mutual assessment that has been carried out in the first step in the cycle. Manpower, technical resources, and funding requirements all need to be addressed.

The technology is determined by the assessment of the severity of the IDD endemic. Priority needs to be given to areas and regions with moderate or severe IDD with the technological implications already cited above. This means that resources and technology must be focused. An indicated in Chapter 7, iodized oil is the major technology of proven effectiveness. Injection or oral administration is available. However, the teams and organization already developed in many countries for the Expanded Programme of Immunization (EPI) program could be of great value to an iodized oil injection programme in a region with severe IDD. Population targets and costs can be specified just as in the case of the EPI programme using the public health care system. This opportunity is particularly relevant to Africa where recent EPI programs have had considerable success.

Such a transition has taken place in Nepal where some 2 million injections of iodized oil have been given in 28 remote districts where iodized salt could not be distributed. A single injection of the oil (1.0 ml) provided an adequate supply for prevention of IDD for about four years (Acharya 1987).

In relation to iodized salt, there will be a need for provision of appropriate legislation to ensure community cooperation in production and distribution.

Political decision

As already pointed out, political decision is critical to the authority of a national commission and to the allocation of sufficient resources for a national programme. Political decision in turn often depends on a degree of 'ground swell' in the community or at least perception by politicians that the issue is a significant one to the community. In the case of IDD control this should be readily achieved if effective communication of the IDD message has taken place.

In Indonesia, effective communication to politicians has taken place so that IDD control has been included in the successive Perlitas (5-year plans) since 1974. This is also important from the point of view of international aid. The international agencies in general follow the priorities established by national governments in their health and social planning.

Aid agencies can allocate resources for national IDD control programme only if governments give priority to such programmes. Then appropriate planning documents need to be presented as a follow-up to such a decision so that the international agency can justify the allocation of resources from its funds. Such agencies have to satisfy their auditors in due course.

In these days of strained budgets both at national governmental level and in the international agencies, there is keen competition for funds. The IDD message has to be clearly stated to receive support. The social and economic benefits need to be specified. More data are required on this aspect.

Dr Henry Levin, an economist from Stanford University, had

been advising on this problem as a consultant for the ICCIDD. He points out the various aspects to be considered in such studies:

1. The costs of an IDD control programme compared to the costs of not having an IDD control programme. These are usually 'invisible'—certainly likely to be regarded as invisible by government officials! But once an IDD control programme is initiated, the costs are visible and have to be justified to the Finance Section. The costs of IDD relate to the non-productivity of the significant percentage who are cretins but also the lowered productivity of those suffering from varying degrees of hypothyroidism. The correction of iodine deficiency leads to restoration of normal thyroid function with improvements in work output and school performance. It also leads to improvements in the productivity of the livestock industry where sheep, cattle or goats are a significant component of agriculture in the particular country.

2. Then there is the question of the particular alternative strategies to be employed in the IDD control programme. The costs of salt iodization would be anticipated to be less than iodized oil but this needs to be verified in relation to the particular country and circumstances of the salt industry. The prospect of salt iodization may be severely curtailed as in Java because of the myriad of small salt producers with salt pans along the North Java Coast. This indicates the desirability of iodized oil if available at reasonable cost.

3. Finally there is the question of the costs and benefits of an IDD control programme compared to other public health programmes. This may be difficult to determine. However the considerable social and economic benefits from the modest expenditure of IDD control programmes make them an attractive alternative.

Implementation

Once a political decision is made on a national IDD control programme with appropriate allocation of resources, implementation can proceed according to the plan that has been submitted. This will involve discussion and coordination with the various sections of the health department (nutrition, family planning, mental health, and the EPI programme). Training programmes will be required for the staff. Purchases of iodized oil, and arrangements for the production and distribution of iodized salt will need to be made. Targets will need to be set for the implementation so that it can be assessed by progress reports.

An example of implementation of a national programme are the recent developments in Peru: in Peru, a situational analysis was carried out by Dr Eduard Pretell and his team. It revealed the following:

(1) iodine deficiency existed in the Sierra and Jungle Regions;
(2) about 50 per cent of the Peruvian population lived in these two areas, accounting for about 9 million inhabitants, of whom approximately 22 per cent were women of fertile age and 12 per cent were children below the age of 14;
(3) a random survey showed that in about 80 per cent of villages the mean urinary excretion of iodine was 100 μg/day or less, and 50 μg/day or less in about 50 per cent of villages;
(4) consequently, the population at risk for IDD would comprise about 7 million inhabitants; and
(5) high prevalences of goitre and of both neurological and myxoedematous cretinism were demonstrated in some surveys (Pretell 1987)

The relation of iodized salt to the situation was as follows:

(1) iodized salt, by law, is produced and distributed by a state company, EMSAL;
(2) only about 30 per cent of iodized salt was reaching the iodine deficient areas and at irregular intervals; its use was very limited or non-existent in the vast majority of villages in these areas; reasons for this included a lack of awareness among the people about the risks of iodine deficiency, inadequate channels of commercialization, high costs, easy accessibility to many sources of non-iodized salt, and ancestral patterns of salt consumption;
(3) a pilot study on the intramuscular administration of iodized oil, started in 1966, demonstrated its effectiveness, not only as a long-lasting means to correct and prevent IDD, but also in convincing people of the beneficial results of iodine treatment within a short period of time.

In due course there followed a demand for iodized salt.

In light of these data, the health authorities of Peru, recognizing the high risks and social cost of IDD and the urgent need for its correction, have taken steps toward the implementation of an effective and aggressive campaign. The first step was to create the Unit for Control of IDD (UCIDD), appointing a minimally sufficient staff of four professionals and four auxiliaries, including two endocrinologists, one epidemiologist, one nutritionist, and one lab technician. The Unit will have the support of a multidisciplinary and multisectoral group representing the Ministries of Education, Agriculture, and Industry, the university system, and the salt industry. The UCIDD will act as a central body located in Lima, the capital of Peru, but its activities will be disseminated to the 57 health areas into which the country is divided. Each health area comprises a group of districts, each with a number of peripheral health services and a hospital.

The second step was the approval of the National Programme to Eradicate Iodine Deficiency Disorders in Peru. The aim of the Programme was to assure adequate iodine for the whole population within two years. This would be followed by the provision of iodized salt for both human and animal consumption within the next 5 to 10 years. The Programme depended on external financial support mainly from the Italian government, (within the framework of the Joint WHO/UNICEF Nutrition Support Programme for Eradication of Endemic Goitre and Cretinism in the Countries of the Andean Region). UNICEF provided important additional support in terms of iodized oil and supplies for its administration; USAID also contributed.

Monitoring and evaluation

Monitoring is concerned with 'process'—the iodized salt production, oil distribution, and details of training programmes.

Evaluation is concerned with 'outcome'—the control of IDD, as indicated by control of iodine deficiency, reduced goitre prevalence reduced prevalence of cretinism, improved school performance, or increased productivity.

An example of monitoring is provided by India, where production of iodated salt had fallen far behind the targets set; only 100 000 tonnes per year (one quarter of the target) were being produced in 1983. This led to a complete reorganization of production with an increase to 500 000 tonnes in 1986 (see Chapter 12).

An example of evaluation is provided by Indonesia. (Dulberg *et*

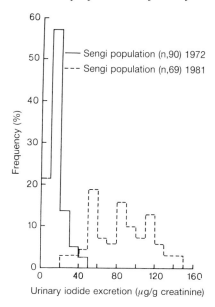

Fig. 8.4. Effect of iodized salt and iodized oil program in Central Java. Severe iodine deficiency was indicated by low urine excretion in 1972 with 7 per cent rate of cretinism (n is the number of subjects tested in each year). In 1981 an evaluation indicated that a normal urine iodine (interrupted line) was associated with total prevention of cretinism since 1974, when the programme began. (From Hetzel 1984, with permission.)

al. 1983). After the introduction of the National Control Programme in 1974 in which both iodized salt and iodized oil were used, an assessment was made in a village community in Central Java in 1981. This revealed an increase in urine iodine excretion to a normal range by comparison with 1972 (Fig. 8.4). Cretinism was no longer found in children under the age of 7, i.e. those children born since 1974 when iodization was introduced, in contrast to a 7 per cent incidence in children in the age range 7–16. These data document the effectiveness of the National Control Programme in one local community, which was studied intensively. In other areas, persistence of goitre indicated inadequate correction of the deficiency (see Chapter 12).

Monitoring and evaluation in Nepal

Another example of the monitoring and evaluation of a national IDD control programme is provided by Nepal (Acharya 1987). Nepal has a population of 15 million, an area of 800 × 160 km, and can be divided into the low level Terai in the south, the high mountains in the north (elevation over 3000 m), and the hilly region in between, with a height from 300–3000 m. A survey in the late 1960s in 19 representative villages showed a significant prevalence of goitre in all areas and an overall prevalence of 55 per cent. In a 1969 survey of two widely separated villages, the goitre prevalence was 74–100 per cent. Cretinism and other developmental anomalies, a low content of iodine in the water and in urine (22 μg/g creatinine), and an elevated radio-iodine uptake were frequent. A survey in 1976 found a goitre prevalence of 55.3 per cent in the Langtang area.

The control strategy consisted of two components, iodated salt and iodized oil by injection. Virtually all Nepal's salt comes from India and is supposed to arrive iodated at 25 parts per million (ppm). It may take two weeks to arrive in Nepal, and may be stored for up to six months before distribution. Many persons from small villages come once a year in the summer to the Terai, and buy salt there to last them for the next year. Collection of salt samples from consumers and retailers shows that most salt is inadequately iodated. Of 13 samples in the Kathmandu Valley, only five had values of 15 ppm or more. In other sampling elsewhere in Nepal, the majority of samples had less than the desired 15 ppm.

An iodized oil programme was initiated in 1979 to provide prophylaxis while waiting for an effective iodated salt programme. Thus far it has covered 28 remote northern districts of the country in which iodized salt is unavailable. Since 1981 more than 2 million people have been injected. In each district a preliminary survey was done to estimate goitre prevalence. Teams of two vaccinators each went systematically through the district giving iodized oil, 0.5 ml to children below one year and 1 ml to others. Each team was expected to administer at least 50 injections per day, which would allow approximately 11 000 injections per team per year.

Communication efforts consisted of posters, flash cards, and radio spots. Prior to an injection campaign, workshops were conducted for community leaders.

Problems have included: administrative and logistic difficulties;

lack of community awareness because of high illiteracy; inadequate baseline information; failure to use alternative interventions; inadequate monitoring of salt iodation; and lack of follow-up data on the impact of iodized oil programmes. A follow-up survey was conducted in 1985 with two objectives: to determine the severity of IDD in representative parts of the country, and to determine the impact of iodized oil injection programmes and the optimal time and dose for repeat injection. Survey items included goitre size, hypothyroidism, cretinism, urinary iodine/creatinine ratios, and serum thyroxine and TSH. Some data from individual districts are shown in Table 8.1.

Table 8.1   *Monitoring and evaluation of IDD control in Nepal*

District	Region	*Iodine supplementation*	*Prevalance goitre (%)*	*Urine iodine**
Kathmandu	Kathmandu Valley	No oil given	32	2
Lalitpur	Kathmandu Valley	No oil given	35	5
Bhaktapur	Kathmandu Valley	No oil given	35	3
Nuwakot	Central	Oil 2 years before	32	3
Mustang	Western	Oil 2 years before	50	None
Bajhang	Far Western	Oil 3–4 years before	65	3
Kalikot	Midwestern	Oil 4 years before	63	3
Rasuwa	Central	Oil 5 years before	47	23
Myagdi	Western	No oil given	57	32

From Acharya (1987), with permission.

* % less than 50 μg iodine per g creatinine

It will be seen that the lowest goitre rates are found in the three districts (Kathmandu, Lalitpur and Bhaktapur) in the Kathmandu Valley. The salt iodine levels are higher in two of these districts. However, it would seem likely that increased iodine intake due to diet diversification is also playing a significant role in the reduced goitre prevalence. This would be likely to occur as a biproduct of tourism. In the next two districts (Nuwakot and Mustang) iodized oil injections had been given two years before, with some control of goitre. In Bajlang and Kalikot, oil had been given 3–4 years before; goitre rates were high in spite of an adequate level of urine iodine excretion. In Myagdi, the most remote district in an inaccessible valley, which had not received iodized oil, the goitre rate was 57 per cent, 28 cretins were seen in one village, and the urine iodine excretion was much lower. Salt iodine levels were very low (2–4 ppm) in Myagdi, Kalikot, and Bajhang, which indicated the difficulties of transportation.

Conclusions from this evaluation were:

1. An iodized oil injection (1 ml) lasted approximately 4 years.
2. Oil injections should be repeated in those districts previously injected. Oral administration could also be used.
3. The salt iodization program needed strengthening. Five iodated salt plants are proposed at the points of import from India.
4. An iodine laboratory should be established in Kathmandu.

Conclusion

Monitoring and evaluation are essential for iodization programme to ensure quantitative correction of iodine deficiency. Iodized oil is indicated when there is doubt about salt iodization. Iodized oil makes eradication of IDD possible.

The details of implementation will inevitably vary by country and by region within a country. Target populations need to be specified and sampled before the programme and then monitored afterwards. The extent of population covered by the programmes, by comparison with the total iodine deficient populations, will give some indication of the gap that still has to be met. These various steps are all quite feasible and practicable, and are essential to eradication of IDD, one definite target for the year 2000.

Bibliography

Acharya, S. (1987). Monitoring and evaluation of an IDD control program in Nepal. In *The prevention and control of iodine deficiency disorders* (eds. B. S. Hetzel, J. T. Dunn, and J. B. Stanbury) pp. 213–18. Elsevier, Amsterdam.

Dulberg, E. M., Widjaja, Djokomoeljanto, R., Hetzel, B. S., and Belmont, L. (1983). Evaluation of the iodization program in Central Java with reference to the prevention of endemic cretinism and motor coordination defects. In *Current problems in thyroid research* (eds. Ui, Torizuka,

Nagataki, and Miyai). International Congress Series 605, pp. 394–7. Excerpta Medica Amsterdam.

Dunn, J.T., Pretell, E.A., Daza, C.H., and Viteri, F.E. (eds.) (1986). *Towards the eradication of endemic goiter, cretinism, and iodine deficiency*. Scientific Publication No. 502. PAHO, Washington.

Follis, R.H. (1964). Recent studies in iodine malnutrition and endemic goitre. *Medical Clinics of North America* **48**, 1919–24.

Hetzel, B.S. (1987). An overview of the prevention and control of iodine deficiency disorders. In *The prevention and control of iodine deficiency disorders* (eds. B.S. Hetzel, J.T. Dunn, and J.B. Stanbury) pp. 7–31. Elsevier, Amsterdam.

Levin, H.M. (1987). Economic dimensions of iodine deficiency disorders. In *The prevention and control of iodine deficiency disorders* (eds. B.S. Hetzel, J.T. Dunn, and J.B. Stanbury) pp. 195–208. Elsevier, Amsterdam.

MacLennan, R. and Gaitan, E. Measurement of thyroid size in epidemiologic surveys. In *Endemic goiter and cretinism: continuing threats to world health* (eds. J.T. Dunn and G.A. Medeiros-Neto). PAHO Scientific Publication 292, pp. 195–7. Pan American Health Organization, Washington, DC 1974.

Manoff, R.K. (1987). Social marketing; new tool to combat iodine deficiency disorders. In *The prevention and control of iodine deficiency disorders* (eds. B.S. Hetzel, J.T. Dunn, and J.B. Stanbury) pp. 165–175. Elsevier, Amsterdam.

Perez, C., Scrimshaw, N.S. and Munoz, J.A. Technique of endemic goitre surveys. In *Endemic goitre*, World Health Organization, Monograph Series No. 44, pp. 369–83. Geneva, 1960.

Pretell, E.A. (1987). The national IDD control program in Peru: Implementation of a model. In *The prevention and control of iodine deficiency disorders* (eds. B.S. Hetzel, J.T. Dunn, and J.B. Stanbury) pp. 209–12. Elsevier, Amsterdam.

Further Reading

IDD Newsletter. Vol. 3 (2), May 1987.

Manoff, R.K. (1985) *Social marketing: new imperative for public health*. Praeger, New York.

Manoff, R.K. (1987). Social marketing: new tool to combat iodine deficiency disorders. In *The prevention and control of iodine deficiency disorders* (eds. B.S. Hetzel, J.T. Dunn, and J.B. Stanbury) pp. 165–75. Elsevier, Amsterdam.

9

International action

It is now clear that large populations are at risk of IDD as a result of living in iodine deficient environments. Iodine deficient environments include the major mountainous regions of the world—the Alps, the Andes, the Himalayas, and the vast mountain ranges of China. The iodine deficiency arises as the result of loss of iodine from the soil as a consequence of leaching by glaciation, snow-water, or high rainfall falling on steep slopes. However, iodine deficiency also occurs in low-lying areas subject to flooding, as in the cases of the Ganges Valley in India and the valley of the Songhua River in North Eastern China (Heilongjiang Province). Here periodic floods leach the soil of iodine. The effect of the deficient soil is simply that all food grown in it will lack iodine. This means that although the food supply may be adequate in terms of energy (or calories) there is a risk of IDD in direct proportion to the severity of the deficiency.

The major iodine deficient areas in the developing countries of the world are shown in Fig. 9.1. It will be seen that there are vast areas in China, India, South-east Asia, and South America following major mountain ranges. The scattered areas in Africa are hilly and mountainous regions as well as the elevated plateau of Southern Africa.

Table 9.1 *Prevalence of iodine deficiency disorders in developing countries and numbers of persons at risk (in millions)*

	At risk	Goitre	Overt cretinism
South-east Asia	280	100	1.5
Asia (other countries)	400	30	0.9
Africa	60	30	0.5
Latin America	60	30	0.25
	800	190	3.15

From WHO and Hetzel (1987), with permission.

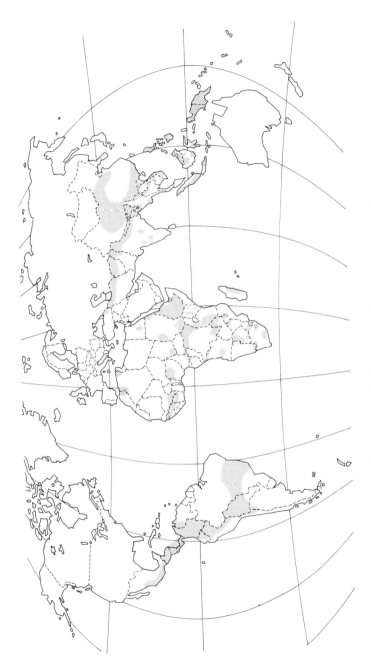

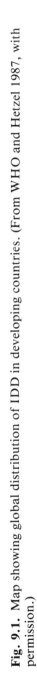

Fig. 9.1. Map showing global distribution of IDD in developing countries. (From WHO and Hetzel 1987, with permission.)

An estimate of the total populations living in these regions and therefore at risk of IDD is shown in Table 9.1. A total of 800 million is estimated to be at risk with nearly a quarter (190 million) suffering from goitre and in excess of 3 million suffering overt cretinism. However, as pointed out in Chapter 5, there are many more suffering lesser degrees of defect and some loss of mental and physical energy from the effect of hypothyroidism. Goitre and cretinism are the visible tip of an 'iceberg' of varying degrees of disability. Iodine deficiency is now seen to be a major impediment to human development (see Chapter 6).

Most people in these regions are living in subsistence agriculture systems. All the food they eat is grown in the local soil and iodine deficiency will persist until iodine comes in either through diversification of the diet or by an iodine supplement. In general, diversification of the diet depends on the development of a cash economy. This is what occurred in the mountainous areas of southern Europe in the earlier decades of the 20th century when goitre and cretinism spontaneously receded without a formal iodine supplementation programme. Diet diversification has also been a major factor in the fall in goitre prevalence in most Western countries, so that by now the condition has almost disappeared with or without iodine supplements. As we shall see (Chapter 10) goitre and cretinism persist in some of the remote areas of Europe, e.g. Sicily, and goitre alone is still widely prevalent in hilly and mountainous areas of Italy and Germany. The increase in iodine intake due to diet diversification is apparently not great enough in these areas to correct the deficiency in the local food supply.

However, in most severely iodine deficient areas of the Third World, vast populations are 'locked into' a system of subsistence agriculture which means that severe IDD will persist. Iodine supplements in some form will be necessary to prevent it.

As we have seen, iodine supplementation is feasible and effective. So the question then arises as to whether we can contemplate a programme of action that would lead to the prevention and control of IDD on a global scale. Can we in fact contemplate elimination of IDD for the Third World just as has occurred for the Western world? We can anticipate some 'spontaneous' improvement in the situation in the less severely affected areas as a result of economic development. Yet for other large populations no such relief is in sight. To control IDD requires effective action for many millions in a number of different countries, most of which have a low average income.

This definition of the problem leads directly to the question of action at the international level involving the United Nations Agencies such as the World Health Organization and UNICEF.

International action

There have in fact been a number of calls for the eradication of IDD by international organizations beginning with the World Food Council in 1974. The list over the period 1974–1983 includes the General Assembly of the United Nations (December 1978) and the International Nutrition Congress (Rio de Janiero, 1978). Subsequently, the Regional WHO/UNICEF Committee for South-East Asia (1981, 1982), the Asia and Oceania Thyroid Congress (Tokyo, 1982), the 4th Asian Congress of Nutrition (Bangkok, 1983), and the Pan American Health Organization (1983) have all followed with similar recommendations.

It is, however, disappointing to record that little happened over the decade 1974–1983 in response to these various resolutions. This clearly reflects the lack of urgency seen for the problem in the midst of competing pressures for other more urgent Third World health problems, including infectious diseases (smallpox, measles, diphtheria, whooping cough, tetanus, polio) and the diarrhoeal diseases.

At the same time, the WHO triumph of the eradication of smallpox encouraged some of us interested in other major global health problems, to think of the eradication of other conditions such as the nutrition disorders due to iodine and Vitamin A deficiency. However, certain conditions had to be met to make such a positive approach possible. These conditions included the following:

(1) that the problem was of significant magnitude to justify a major allocation of resources;
(2) that there were effective preventive measures suitable for use on a mass scale;
(3) that there was an available delivery system; and
(4) that there were practical methods for monitoring and surveillance of the programme so that it could be shown to be effective.

Certainly as long as the problem of iodine deficiency was simply characterized as 'goitre' (or a 'cosmetic' problem) there was not much chance of it receiving attention. The broader concept of the iodine deficiency disorders has been successful in securing much more attention to the problem, at global, regional, and national levels.

There was a good case for support of an international effort similar to that already mounted for smallpox and currently being carried out in relation to child immunization for control of the common childhood infections. This led me to propose the objective of eradication of IDD at the 2nd Asia and Oceania Thyroid Association meeting in Tokyo (1982) and at the 4th Asian Congress of Nutrition (Bangkok 1983). In 1984 this led to an invitation from the Standing Committee on Nutrition (SCN) of the Administrative Coordinating Committee (ACC) of the United Nations Agencies* through the Australian Government to prepare a state of the art review of IDD and the possibility of successful prevention and control. The Report was submitted to the ACC/SCN office in Rome in February 1985.

The International Council for Control of Iodine Deficiency Disorders

In my report I noted the great delay in the application of knowledge to the needs of the millions suffering needlessly. To help bridge this gap I proposed that an expert consultative group of scientists and others able to assist in the development of IDD control programmes be established. Similar groups already existed in relation to two other major nutritional problems: the International Vitamin A Consultative Group (IVACG), and the International Nutritional Anaemia Consultative Group (INACG). They were established around 1975 with support from the US Agency for International Development (USAID).

*This Subcommittee is composed of representatives of the United Nations, the United Nations Development Program (UNDP), the United Nations Environment Program (UNEP), the United Nations Children's Fund (UNICEF), The World Food Council (WFC), The International Fund for Agricultural Development (IFAD), International Labour Office (ILO), Food and Agriculture Organization (FAO), United Nations Education and Social Organization (UNESCO), the World Bank, The World Health Organization (WHO). Representatives of the governments of Australia, Canada, Denmark, Federal Republic of Germany, the Netherlands, Norway, Sweden, Switzerland, the United Kingdom and the USA regularly attend its meetings.

The decision to establish the International Council for Control of Iodine Deficiency Disorders (ICCIDD) was made in Delhi in March 1985, when a group of about ten consultants and advisors was attending the WHO/UNICEF Intercountry Workshop on the Control of IDD in South-east Asia. The decision was made effective by the generous support of UNICEF, which provided a grant of US $150 000 for the first two years. This has now been increased to US $250 000 per year with generous support from the Italian Government. The Australian Government followed with a grant of US $17 000 and subsequently US $25 000 in the second year for the support of the Secretariat in Adelaide, Australia. This grant has now been raised to US $100 000 per year for 2 years (1987–88 and 1988–89).

A series of meetings was held in Delhi in March 1985 and the following aims and objectives were adopted:
(1) promotion of awareness that the IDD problem can be eradicated at an affordable cost;
(2) promotion of assessment of prevalence of IDD in different regions of the world;
(3) the development of strategies for the control and eradication of IDD;
(4) the evaluation of the effectiveness of these strategies;
(5) research on problems related to the control and eradication of IDD;
(6) provision of training programmes; and
(7) maintenance of a panel of expert consultants.

Functions would include:

(1) promotion of the eradication of IDD through scientific meetings, the media, and publications;
(2) consultation as required, and initially meeting at least once per year;
(3) convening working groups on urgent, operational, scientific, and technical issues for international agencies, national governments with major IDD problems, and countries providing bilateral aid for IDD control programmes;
(4) organizing yearly global reviews of progress in eradication of IDD;
(5) sponsoring state of the art reports;
(6) facilitating technical developments (e.g. monitoring labora-

tories, production of iodized salt and oil);

(7) arranging appropriate training of professionals and technologists; and

(8) arranging short-term study visits to exchange experience and
knowledge.

In Kathmandu, Nepal (March 1986), a constitution was adopted
by a Founding Board and office bearers appointed as required by
the Constitution. The ICCIDD has been registered as an international non-profit organization in the State of South Australia and
I have been designated as Public Officer.

The Founding Board   The Board has 32 members of whom 17 are
from less developed countries, 9 are from developed countries, and
5 are employees of international agencies (UNICEF, WHO, and
the World Bank). Professional disciplines represented on the Board
include public health, epidemiology, internal medicine, paediatrics,
community health, economics, communications, endocrinology,
nutrition, salt manufacturing, and health administration. All
members recognize that IDD is a problem involving a number of
different specialties and that the Board requires a multidisciplinary
composition as well as a global distribution.

Current members of the Board are:

EXECUTIVE COMMITTEE: J.B. Stanbury (USA) (Chairman);
V. Ramalingaswami (India) (Vice Chairman); B.S. Hetzel (Australia)
(Executive Director); J.T. Dunn (USA) (Secretary); T. Ma (China);
G. Medeiros-Neto (Brazil); C. Thilly (Belgium).

REGIONAL COORDINATORS: African Region—O.L. Ekpechi
(Nigeria); American Region—E.A. Pretell (Peru); European
Region—F. Delange (Belgium); Middle Eastern Region—M.
Benmiloud (Algeria); South-east Asia Region—C.S. Pandav (India);
Western Pacific Region—T. Ma (China).

OTHER MEMBERS: A. Berg (World Bank); G. Bertolaso (Italy);
R. Carriere (UNICEF); B.A. Charania (Pakistan), N. Chawla
(India); G.A. Clugston (WHO/SEARO); M.C. De Blanco
(Venezuela); R. DeLong (USA); P. Greaves (UNICEF); E.
DeMaeyer (WHO); R. Djokomoeljanto (Indonesia); M.H. Gabr
(Egypt); F.P. Kavishe (Tanzania); N. Kochupillai (India); D.
Lantum (Cameroon); T.Z. Lu (China); V. Mannar (India); R.
Manoff (USA); A. Pradilla (WHO); I. Tarwotjo (Indonesia); F. van
der Haar (The Netherlands).

The ICCIDD already has a global, multidisciplinary network of more than 300 members. These include scientists, planners, communicators, salt technologists, clinical chemists, and other disciplines concerned with IDD control. A Registry of members will be published in due course.

A group of senior advisers has also been appointed in recognition of outstanding services in research and practice in the field of IDD.

The ICCIDD has adopted several strategies in order to achieve its major aim of bridging the knowledge-application gap:

1. *Consultations with international agencies such as WHO and UNICEF, at both global and regional level.* A recent consultation was held with Mr James Grant and senior UNICEF staff in New York (September 1985). This led to important initiatives including the development of a crash IDD control programme in Southern Peru. At the regional level a Joint WHO/UNICEF/ICCIDD Regional Seminar took place at Yaounde, Cameroon, March 1987 to develop a regional strategy for IDD control in Africa. In addition, consultations have taken place at country level (Bolivia, Nepal, Indonesia, and India).

2. *Publications.* These include the *IDD Newsletter*, edited by Dr John Dunn, a quarterly publication providing a comprehensive review of IDD related activities, regional reports, and regular review of the scientific literature. In addition the ICCIDD has a programme for the publication of monographs. It subsidized the publication of the proceedings of the two satellite meetings held before the 9th International Thyroid Conference in São Paulo, Brazil (August, 1985) under the title *Iodine deficiency disorders and congenital hypothyroidism.* Its first major activity has been the publication of a monograph on *The prevention and control of the iodine deficiency disorders* which appeared early in 1987. Other publications are required such as manuals on goitre surveys, iodized salt production, and laboratory methods for the determination of iodine which are now in the course of preparation.

3. *Working groups on particular problems.* At this stage there are four designated working groups: communication, economics, iodized oil, and iodized salt.

4. *Regional activities through the regional coordinators.* These include:

(1) the development of links with country governments, and international agencies at regional level, designed to help with effective IDD control programmes;

(2) assistance in providing information on all aspects of IDD control programmes;

(3) assistance in the organization of country or regional level training programmes and workshops on IDD control;

(4) development of a multidisciplinary team available to act as an expert resource for the development of IDD control programmes;

(5) development of regional and country level publications on various aspects of IDD control.

Apart from these and other specific strategies the ICCIDD is able to take up the general task of advocacy of IDD control programmes. This it can do by lobbying international agencies and governments. It can help to broaden the constituency for support of IDD control to include journalists, chambers of commerce, consumer groups, unions and employer groups, as well as professional bodies. The ICCIDD could also function as an 'Amnesty International for IDD'. Such a function cannot readily be carried out by WHO because of its existing relationships with country governments. The ICCIDD can also act as an 'honest broker' in being willing to link up donors with countries and programmes. All these suggestions are being actively pursued by the Executive and Board.

In the meantime IDD is being incorporated into the WHO/UNICEF Child Survival and Development Revolution (CSDR) Programme along with child immunization, and oral rehydration therapy for diarrhoea, and breast feeding (Cash *et al.* 1987). (See concluding part of this book.)

The World Health Assembly 1986

The World Health Assembly meets every year at the World Health Organization Headquarters in Geneva. It is attended by member states, with delegations led by ministers of health and heads of health departments. It is the Health 'Parliament' of the world. 166 countries are members. The deliberations are organized by an Executive Board which is elected from the member states' representatives every two years.

The deliberations in recent years have been affected by the

political polarization that has occurred with the strong positions taken up by the 120 non-aligned countries. Certain intractable political situations are brought up for discussion such as the plight of the Palestinian refugees, which does have health implications. These can lead to prolonged debates. However, the World Health Assembly is a most important body in developing policies in the field of international health.

In May 1986 at the 39th World Health Assembly, Australia sponsored a Resolution on the Prevention and Control of Iodine Deficiency Disorders as follows:

The Thirty-Ninth World Health Assembly,

- Noting the high prevalence of iodine deficiency disorders, affecting more than 400 million people in Asia alone as well as millions in Africa and South America;
- Concerned that iodine deficiency disorders include not only goitrous enlargement of the thyroid gland but also stillbirths, abortions and congenital anomalies; endemic cretinism characterised most commonly by mental deficiency, deaf mutism and spastic diplegia and lesser degrees of neurological defect related to fetal iodine deficiency; and impaired mental function in children and adults with reduced levels of circulating thyroxine;
- Aware that low cost effective technology, including use of iodized salt and iodized oil (by injection or mouth), is available for the prevention and control of iodine deficiency disorders;
- Considering that prevention and eradication of iodine deficiency disorders, which will result in improved quality of life, and productivity, and improved educability of children and adults suffering from iodine deficiency disorders, is feasible within the next 5–10 years;
- Aware that the United Nations Administrative Committee on Coordination's Sub-Committee on Nutrition had called for a global strategy by governments and United Nations agencies to prevent and control iodine deficiency disorders; and that this recommendation had been endorsed by the Administrative Committee on Coordination for immediate and high priority action;

1. Urges all member states to give high priority to the prevention and control of iodine deficiency disorders, wherever these problems exist, through appropriate nutritional programs as part of primary health care;
2. Requests the Director-General
(1) to give all possible support to member states, as and when requested, in

assessing the most appropriate approaches in the light of national circumstances, needs, and resources, to preventing and controlling iodine deficiency disorders;

(2) to collaborate with member states in the monitoring of the incidence and prevalence of iodine deficiency disorders;

(3) to prepare suitable materials for adaptation and use at national level for training health and development workers in the early identification and treatment of iodine deficiency disorders and the implementation of appropriate public health preventive programs in iodine deficient areas;

(4) to coordinate with other intergovernmental agencies and appropriate nongovernmental agencies, the launching and management of intensive and extensive international action to combat iodine deficiency disorders including the mobilization of financial and other resources required for such actions;

(5) to report to the World Health Assembly on progress in this area, including the financial aspects.

The Resolution was proposed by Australia and co-sponsored by the following 22 countries—

Belgium	India	Republic of Korea
Bhutan	Indonesia	Romania
Bulgaria	Mexico	Sweden
Cameroon	Nepal	United Kingdom
Chile	New Zealand	Vietnam
China	Nigeria	Yugoslavia
Finland	Philippines	
France	Poland	

The Resolution was carried unanimously. It is a major step forward for all members of the ICCIDD and others concerned with IDD control. A 10-year programme of work for the prevention and control of IDD has now been drawn up by the Standing Committee of Nutrition of the Administrative Coordinating Committee of the United Nations Agencies (the ACC/SCN). The ICCIDD has been recognized by the Chairman of the ACC/SCN (Dr Abraham Horwitz) as the expert consultative group for this programme.

As the Director-General of the World Health Organization (Dr H. Mahler) pointed out in his message to the inaugural meeting of the ICCIDD, 'If IDD is under control in the majority of industrialized countries, as well as in some developing ones, much remains to be accomplished in Africa and in many parts of Asia, the

Pacific and South America. Immediate action is called for on a number of fronts: improved prevalence assessments; definitions of control methods and prevention strategies; education of the public; motivation of health authorities and training of health personnel; drafting and adoption of appropriate health legislation; and establishment of effective monitoring and evaluation measures.

Technical and financial resources, while an obvious prerequisite to providing the support governments need, are only part of the answer; even large sums of money alone would be powerless to meet the needs of potential beneficiaries who fail to understand the risks they and their offspring face or who are insufficiently motivated to take the steps necessary to overcome them.

The International Council for Control of Iodine Deficiency Disorders can play an important role in this regard, and WHO looks forward to tapping its considerable technical expertise and experience, both in helping it to support countries develop sound prevention and control programs and in conducting needed research leading to advances in this field.'

A global strategy for the prevention and control of iodine deficiency disorders: proposal for a ten-year programme of support for countries

In October 1985, the Administrative Coordinating Committee (ACC) of the United Nations decided that priority attention be given to the prevention and control of IDD. The ACC through its subcommittee on nutrition (SCN) then requested the World Health Organization to prepare 'A global strategy for the Prevention and Control of IDD: Proposal for a Ten Year Program of Support to Countries'. This report was duly completed in August 1986, and sent out for review and comments by the other UN agencies, experts and others with particular knowledge. The Report was then redrafted and finally submitted to the 13th Session of the ACC/SCN held in Washington 2–6 March 1987. The representatives of the various UN agencies (WHO, FAO, UNICEF, UNU and the World Bank) indicated their support for the ten-year programme and requested the Chairman to forward the proposal to the ACC and so to the Secretary General of the United Nations. The Report points out that:

In developing countries alone, 800 million persons are at risk from IDD, which include goitre, endemic cretinism and lesser degrees of neurological defects, and impaired mental function in children and adults. Of this number some 190 million have goitre . . . Undisputed evidence shows that IDD can be successfully and inexpensively prevented and controlled, and that a reduction of goitre rates to below 10 per cent is entirely feasible within a decade. The prevention and control of IDD, because of its dramatic impact on the quality of life, productivity and educability of millions, would make a significant contribution to attaining the goal of health for all by the year 2000 . . . Firm commitment and close cooperation—on the part of governments, organizations and bodies of the United Nations system, government-sponsored bilateral development agencies, and interested non-governmental organizations—are essential ingredients for its success.

A Working Group was established which includes representatives of UN agencies directly involved in the programme, interested bilateral agencies, and ICCIDD. A major role of the Working Group is to identify financial resources for the development of the programme and to:

(1) monitor the prevalence and severity of IDD;
(2) facilitate the launching of programmes for the control of IDD;
(3) help mobilize international resources to support such programmes;
(4) monitor progress of IDD control programmes;
(5) report to the ACC/SCN on progress.

The first meeting was held at the PAHO office in Washington on 6th March 1987. The Executive Director of the ICCIDD was appointed Secretary of the group and was asked to convene meetings in consultation with an appointed Chairman from one of the UN agencies. The first Chairman appointed was Dr Peter Greaves of UNICEF. It was agreed that all bilateral countries represented on the ACC/SCN should receive a copy of the IDD Working Group frame of reference with an invitation to them to consider support for the ten-year programme when approached.

So far four countries (Italy, Canada, Sweden, and The Netherlands) have indicated their interest in the support of national IDD control programmes.

The next four chapters review the present status of IDD and IDD control in four major regions of the world—Europe, largely under control; Latin America, some progress but still needing true commitment in many countries; Asia, with the challenge of massive iodine deficient populations; and Africa, where little has been done so far.

Conclusion

Notable recent international action has taken place for the global control of IDD. There have been three major developments:

(1) the World Health Assembly's resolution of 1986 requesting the Director General of WHO to give all possible support to member States, and expressing the view that significant progress in prevention and control was feasible within the next 5–10 years;

(2) the establishment of the International Council for Control of Iodine Deficiency Disorders (ICCIDD), multidisciplinary group of 300 scientists, planners, and public health administrators who have expertise relevant to national IDD control programmes;

(3) the adoption of a global strategy for the prevention and control of IDD involving a 10-year programme of support for countries with major IDD problems, by the Subcommittee of Nutrition of the Administrative Coordinating Committee of the United Nations Agencies.

These three steps are, respectively, political, scientific, and administrative developments which taken together give cause for hope that significant progress in the prevention and control of IDD can be achieved in the next 5–10 years.

Bibliography

Cash, R., Kensch, G. T., and Lamstein, J. (eds). (1987). *Child health and survival*. Croom Helm, London.

Hetzel, B.S. (1985). *Toward a global strategy for the prevention and control of iodine deficiency disorders*. Report to ACC/SCN, Rome.

Hetzel, B.S. (1987). An overview of the prevention and control of iodine deficiency disorders. In *The prevention and control of iodine deficiency disorders* (ed. B.S. Hetzel, J.T. Dunn, and J.B. Stanbury), pp. 7–31. Elsevier, Amsterdam.

Mahler, H. F. (1987). Message to the inaugural meeting of the International

Council for the control of iodine deficiency disorders. In *The prevention and control of iodine deficiency disorders* (ed. B.S. Hetzel, J.T. Dunn, and J.B. Stanbury), pp. 1–2. Elsevier, Amsterdam.

United Nations Administrative Coordinating Committee Sub-Committee on Nutrition. (1987). *A global strategy for the prevention and control of iodine deficiency disorders: proposal for a ten-year program of support to countries.* Rome.

World Health Organization (1986). *Report of the 39th World Health Assembly.* Resolution 29. Geneva.

Further Reading

Hetzel, B.S., Dunn, J.T., and Stanbury, J.B. (eds.). (1987). *The prevention and control of iodine deficiency disorders.* Elsevier, Amsterdam.

PART III

The present challenge: A massive global problem

10

Europe

Chapter 2 reviewed the history of goitre and cretinism in Europe. The people affected were mainly those living in the Alpine region which included Switzerland, Northern Italy, and Austria. The early descriptions came from this region; goitre and cretinism have been part of the human landscape for many centuries as recorded in art and literature long before scientific observations were made.

Towards the end of the 19th century and into the 20th century a definite decline in goitre and cretinism was reported from these countries. This is indicated by data from the examination of army recruits, schoolchildren, and other groups. Spontaneous decline in cretinism was reported in Switzerland, Italy, and Yugoslavia prior to the distribution of iodized salt. However, the distribution of iodized salt greatly accelerated this process as was seen in Switzerland.

These reports had given rise to the impression that the problem of IDD in Europe was no longer significant. It was therefore a considerable surprise to read a comprehensive report (Scriba *et al.* 1985) on goitre and iodine deficiency in Europe, published by a special committee of the European Thyroid Association in the *Lancet*, which indicated that IDD was still a serious problem in a number of countries.

The present status of IDD and its control in Europe

The European Committee reviewed available information from each country by reference to epidemiological studies, reports from individuals, and by questionnaires to health departments. They found there was a lack of epidemiological data in many European countries, but enough data were available to give some idea of the situation.

Goitre prevalence in various countries is shown on the map (Fig. 10.1). The figures are based on samples varying in number

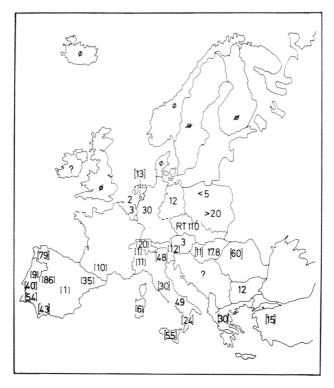

Fig. 10.1. Goitre prevalence in percent by country. Regional values are denoted by brackets. (From Scriba *et al*. 1985, with permission.)

from a few hundred to several hundred thousand. High figures are shown for the Federal Republic of Germany, Italy, Greece, Turkey, Bulgaria, and Spain. The four Scandinavian countries, Norway, Sweden, Finland, and Denmark, have virtually no goitre. In general the goitre prevalence increases from northern to southern Europe.

Data from determination of urine iodine excretion reveals, as would be expected, an inverse association between the goitre prevalence and urine iodine levels. The available data are shown in fig. 10.2. There is a striking contrast between the data from the three Scandinavian countries, Norway, Sweden, and Finland, which report a urine iodine excretion of 200–500 µg/dl in contrast to the Federal Republic of Germany with a country level of 60 µg/dl.

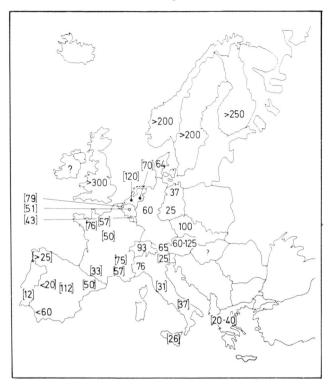

Fig. 10.2. Urinary iodine excretion in micrograms iodine per gram creatinine; regional values denoted by brackets. (From Scriba *et al*. 1985, with permission.)

We will now review IDD in Europe by reference to the two major categories of data that are available:

(1) *goitre prevalence*, and
(2) *data from newborn infants*.

Recent goitre prevalence in Europe

The European countries have been divided into three groups in the Report (Scriba *et al*. 1985). They are:

(1) countries which are now free of endemic goitre;
(2) countries showing persistence of endemic goitre;
(3) an intermediate group.

No information was available from Albania, France, or the USSR.

(1) *Countries free of endemic goitre*   This group included Norway, Sweden, and Finland, and probably Denmark, Iceland, the United Kingdom, and Ireland. Finland has had a particularly successful programme of salt iodation which provides a valuable example for other European countries. The increased consumption of iodized salt was promoted actively by the State Commission of Nutrition and the salt iodization programme was combined with a public education campaign.

In Eastern Finland a reduction in goitre rate to about 1 per cent was found compared with 15–30 per cent in the early 1950s. This reduction resulted from a recommended level of 25 mg/kg (previously 10 mg/kg) and greatly increased consumption, so that 75 per cent of the total amount of salt sold in 1969 was iodized compared with less than 50 per cent in 1959. There was also evidence of increased levels of urinary iodine excretion (less than 45–60 μg/d in 1959 compared with 200 μg/d in 1969). It is possible that other dietary changes contributed to the increased iodine intake.

In the United Kingdom there is now little evidence of goitre following the earlier well known 'Derbyshire neck', and goitre in other areas. The average iodine intake has been shown to be 323 μg per day due to the high iodine content of milk. This is due mainly to the use of iodophors in the dairy industry (see below).

(2) *Countries showing persistent goitre*   No less than 12 countries have persistent endemic goitre. In Austria, Hungary, Poland, and Yugoslavia there are substantial areas with high goitre prevalence suggesting an ineffective iodized salt programme. Dietary iodine, as indicated by urine iodine measurement, remains low. Analysis of the salt iodine reveals low levels in the range of 4–12 mg of iodine per kilogram of salt. In general, levels in excess of 20 mg/kilo are required to maintain the normal iodine intake of 150–300 μg per day (recommended by the WHO) where there is little or no iodine from other components of the diet.

In Austria there has been a national programme since 1967. Goitre prevalence has fallen in the Tyrol from 46 per cent to 12 per cent in schoolchildren; the rate in army recruits is now 3.3 per cent. However, urine iodine excretion remains low in the Tyrol, Salzburg, Graz, and Vienna. It was concluded that the present level of salt iodization (10 mg KI per kilo) is inadequate.

In another group of countries there is no iodized salt programme.

These include the Federal Republic of Germany, the German Democratic Republic, Greece, Italy, Portugal, Romania, Spain, and Turkey. Goitre is a continuing problem and cretinism can still be found, as in Sicily and Spain. The Report concludes that these countries require IDD control programmes urgently.

In the Federal Republic of Germany there was a goitre prevalence of 15 per cent in a study of 5.4 million military recruits. Evidence of iodine deficiency has been found in children and adults. In the German Democratic Republic there is an overall goitre prevalence of 12 per cent in military recruits.

In Greece there is a 50 per cent prevalence of goitre in some rural areas. The introduction of iodized salt in Athens has increased the urine excretion of iodine by over 100 per cent.

In Italy there is a continued high prevalence of goitre from Sicily (25–80 per cent in schoolchildren), Tuscany (63 per cent in school-children), the Alto-Adige, Lazio and Calabria, and the Apennines. There is only limited availability of iodized salt.

In Spain, a recent survey showed a goitre prevalence of 86 per cent in schoolchildren in the Las Hurdes region (near Salamanca) with persistent cretinism.

(3) *The intermediate group*
Bulgaria, Czechoslovakia, The Netherlands, and Switzerland have had major IDD problems in the past but effective programmes have been implemented so that iodine intake is now adequate. There is some persistence of goitre in older age groups as in Switzerland where a 1975 survey showed a goitre prevalence of 20 per cent in adults aged 20–39 and 60 per cent in the 60–79 age group which reflects the inadequate iodization of salt in earlier decades. The level of salt iodization has been progressively increased in Switzerland since 1955 to the present 20 mg KI per kilogram of salt. A recent survey of army recruits revealed a goitre prevalence of less than 1 per cent.

In the Netherlands, endemic goitre is still present in some regions. IDD control is believed to be inadequate. An increase in bread salt iodide from 46–60 mg KI/k has been recommended to provide 20 μg iodine from each slice of bread. A salt iodide level of 26.2 mg per kilo has also been recommended.

Considerable success with iodine prophylaxis has been reported from Bulgaria and Czechoslovakia. In Bulgaria, iodized salt

(20 mg KI/kg) has led to the elimination of goitre in schoolchildren. In Czechoslovakia, goitre prevalence dropped greatly following the introduction of iodized salt in 1953. Cessation of prophylaxis in two districts led to a rapid fall in urine iodine excretion which indicated the need for continuation of the programme.

Studies in neonates

The importance of the state of thyroid function in the neonate has been emphasized in Part I. At birth the brain of the human infant has only reached about one third of its full size and continues to grow rapidly until the end of the second year. The thyroid hormone, dependent on an adequate supply of iodine, is essential for normal brain development as has been shown from the animal studies described in Chapter 5. Recent European data (Delange *et al.* 1986) confirm that severe iodine deficiency affects neonatal thyroid function and hence is a threat to early brain development.

In Table 10.1 a comparison is made between the incidence of permanent and transient neonatal hypothyroidism in Europe and North America. The rates of permanent hypothyroidism are similar but the rate for transient hypothyroidism is greater in Europe than in North America by a factor of more than seven. Transient hypothyroidism has been reported previously in Europe mainly from areas with a borderline or clearly deficient iodine supply. It has also been shown that this condition can be corrected by iodine supplementation.

Table 10.1 *Comparison of the incidence of permanent and transient primary hypothyroidism in North American and European neonates*

Regions	Number of infants screened	Incidence of primary hypothyroidism	
		permanent	*transient*
North America	1238 247	1/4550	1/61 910
Europe	1276 307	1/3980	1/8260

From Delange *et al.* (1986), with permission.

In these investigations, a direct relation was shown between the urinary iodine excretion and the milk iodine intake. Hence, the urinary iodine excretion can be used as an index of the dietary supply of iodine. Subsequently a series of 1076 urine samples were collected and analysed from 16 centres in 10 different European countries, in addition to a series from Toronto, Canada. The results of these determinations are shown in Table 10.2. The results were expressed in percentiles rather than in arithmetic means. Some very high values were seen which could be attributed to the use of iodized contrast media for radiological investigation of the mother during pregnancy.

Table 10.2 *Frequency distributions of urinary iodine concentrations in healthy full-term infants in 14 European cities and in Toronto, Canada*

| City | Number of infants | Urinary iodine concentration | | | Frequency (%) of values below 5 µg/dl |
		10th percentile	50th percentile	90th percentile	
Toronto	81	4.3	14.8	37.5	11.9
Rotterdam	64	4.5	16.2	33.2	15.3
Helsinki	39	4.8	11.2	31.8	12.8
Stockholm	52	5.1	11.0	25.3	5.9
Catania	14	2.2	7.1	11.0	38.4
Zurich	62	2.6	6.2	12.9	34.4
Lille	82	2.0	5.8	15.2	37.2
Brussels	196	1.7	4.8	16.7	53.2
Rome	114	1.5	4.7	13.8	53.5
Toulouse	37	1.2	2.9	9.4	69.4
Berlin	87	1.3	2.8	13.6	69.7
Göttingen	81	0.9	1.5	4.7	91.3
Heidelberg	39	1.1	1.3	4.0	89.8
Freiburg	41	1.1	1.1	2.3	100.0
Jena	54	0.4	0.8	2.2	100.0

The European cities are listed according to decreasing values of 50th percentile.

From Delange *et al.* (1986), with permission.

There was a marked difference in the results from the various cities. The high levels in Rotterdam, Helsinki, and Stockholm differed from the low levels in Göttingen, Heidelberg, Freiburg, and

Jena by a factor of more than 10. Intermediate levels were seen in Cantania, Zurich, and Lille.

Data on neonatal thyroid function were analysed from four cities where enough newborns (30 000–102 000) had been assayed. The incidence of permanent sporadic hypothyroidism was very similar in the four cities but the rate of transient hypothyroidism was much greater in Freiberg, associated with the lowest level of urine iodine excretion, than in Stockholm, with intermediate findings from Rome and Brussels. These data confirm the significance of low iodine intake for neonatal thyroid function.

Further evidence of iodine deficiency is available from studies in East Germany as observed in Karl Marx Stadt and other regions. (Bauch *et al.* 1986). In 489 pregnant women, 60 per cent had developed goitre. By contrast, 200 pregnant women who were treated with thyroid hormones or with hormones plus iodine showed no significant change in neck size. In the case of the newborns, 12.8 per cent had enlarged thyroids in the range 9.2–45 g in weight. If iodine nutrition was normal, the thyroid weighed less than 3 g.

These data provide strong evidence indicating the need for effective IDD control programmes in those European countries with continuing iodine deficiency, particularly the Federal Republic of Germany and the German Democratic Republic. Now that screening programmes for neonatal hypothyroidism are becoming generally available, the results could be used to assess the adequacy of corrective measures.

At a recent meeting (1988) Professor W. Meng has now reported on the benefits of iodization in the GDR since 1983. There has been a fall in the rate of goitre and neonatal hypothyroidism. There has also been an increase in the productivity of farm animals.

The challenge of IDD control in Europe

The data reviewed in the two previous sections indicate a substantial challenge to a number of governments. A review of the successful control of IDD in Switzerland may provide some useful lessons.

The pioneers in the introduction of iodine prophylaxis in Switzerland were Hunziger, who in 1916 first used iodide tablets in the same way and at the same time as Marine did in Ohio, USA; and Bayard, a local practitioner who first mixed iodized salt in 1918 in the Matterhorn region. Bayard gave it to families who showed regression of goitre after six months; he supported his observations with photographs.

However, it was Dr Hans Eggenberger of the canton of Appenzell who first confronted the political problem of securing community acceptance for iodine prophylaxis. He became convinced of the merit of iodized salt because of his observations, carried out between 1916 and 1920, in the neighbouring cantons of Vaud and Friboorg. Vaud was free of goitre but the immediately adjacent Friboorg had a high prevalence. He determined that the two cantons had different sources of salt. The salt for Friboorg came from the Rhine Saltworks, while that for Vaud came from Bex. He then found that the salt from Bex contained iodine (naturally) but that from the Rhine saltworks did not. This was a 'natural experiment' which indicated to Eggenberger the suitability of salt as a vehicle for iodine prophylaxis.

In February 1922 he organized a petition from the people of his canton of Appenzell. Every man was persuaded to sign. This meant that the canton had to provide iodized salt for all its citizens. Eggenberger began by producing the iodized salt himself at his hospital at Herisau in Appenzell. It was then added to the salt coming in through each railway station from the Rhine Saltworks. The benefits soon became apparent in the drop in goitre prevalence.*

The monitoring of the effect of iodized salt in the 23 cantons of Switzerland was provided by the yearly compulsory examination of new army service recruits. This provided an indisputable indication of the effectiveness of the iodized salt programme. Eventually certain cantons that had lagged in the provision of iodized salt (due to the opposition, in two cases, of their leading surgeons) eventually were forced to adopt the measure.

It is important to note that the cost of iodized salt is the same as non-iodized salt in Switzerland due to a subsidy provided by the cantons. The monitoring of the iodized salt is carried out at cantonal level. All salt added to processed foods by the food industry is iodized, which means that approximately 70 per cent of the intake is covered. Hence the choice of iodized salt for the other 30 per cent is

---

* Information kindly supplied by Dr H.J. Wespi of Aarau, son-in-law of Eggenberger and himself an important contributor to the development and promotion of iodized salt in Switzerland.

not as important as it was in the past when processed foods were not so large a component of the diet.

In considering the relevance of this history for other European countries today, a different social situation must be taken into account. The 'Green' parties are now very active in Europe, especially in Germany (FRG). They are likely to oppose a campaign to add iodine to salt no matter how great are demonstrable benefits because of an obsession with 'natural food'. A carefully designed public education campaign is required for Germany, Italy, and any other countries with such strong 'Green' groups. The concern about the salt content of the diet in relation to hypertension is another factor to be considered but an increase in concentration will readily compensate for a lowered salt intake.

It would seem most expedient for salt iodization to begin in certain regions where IDD is a bigger problem. This could be carefully monitored (by goitre prevalence in schoolchildren, urinary iodine excretion, and if possible blood thyroxine (T_4 levels) in these regions together with other regions where iodized salt was not being used. The difference can then be used to introduce a competitive element between the regions, as occurred in Switzerland between the cantons. The citizens might then respond with more motivation. As acceptance by the regions increases, a national programme could become feasible. However, not all regions are iodine deficient and so the argument for local as opposed to national measures will be brought up.

If there are difficulties with iodized salt, what are the alternatives? There are, as we have already seen in Part II, iodized oil, bread, water, or milk. Of these, the bread, water, and milk raise difficulties for a Green lobby. The occurrence of iodine in milk is often the result of the use of iodophors as disinfectants in the dairy industry. Iodide is also used as a trace element additive for cattle feed in the USA. This has the advantage that milk is more likely to be consumed by children. There has been concern about excessive iodine levels in milk, but this has probably been exaggerated; most Japanese consume 0.5–1.0 mg of iodine per day without any ill affects being demonstrable. However, the continued provision of iodine in milk rests on industrial practice which can easily change.

The use of iodized oil by mouth has the advantage that it is a prescriptive measure that can be introduced through the health care system without legislative provision. Administration to people over the age of 45 can be avoided, and the vulnerable groups of women of child bearing age and children can be targetted specifically by the programme.

IDD in Italy

IDD has been a matter of concern to Italian thyroidologists for several years. The views of this important group have been summarized in the 'Italian Iodine Manifesto' drafted at their National Meeting in Turin in November 1985 and approved by the Italian Society of Endocrinology at its national meeting in Bari, May 1986. It has been widely distributed among physicians, health officials, and political authorities. It was also published in full in the *IDD Newsletter* (November 1986). The last two sections are quoted here:

Iodine deficiency and endemic goitre in Italy
  The existence of large areas of endemic goitre and iodine deficiency in Italy has been described in the past, and confirmed in more recent studies. Foci of endemic goitre have been found throughout the country from the Alps down to the southern Apennines as well as in the islands. Cases of endemic cretinism are still present in the areas of more severe iodine deficiency. Even in the areas apparently spared by endemic goitre, the dietary iodine intake is generally lower than that recommended by WHO. Thus, all the people living in Italy, including the urban areas, are exposed to some degree of iodine deficiency and consequently to the risk of goitre and other IDDs. Early but transient programs of iodine prophylaxis in Italy have been limited to selected areas with a high prevalence of endemic goitre: Val d'Aosta in 1909, Valtellina, and the montane areas of Piedmont and Lombardy in 1925. In 1972 the government authorized the production of iodized salt by the salt plant of the State Monopoly. Its sale was limited to the areas with proved endemic goitre. Such limitation greatly reduced the efficacy of a nationwide iodine prophylaxis. The recognition of this drawback and the abolition of the state monopoly of salt production led to a new law in 1977 liberalizing the production of iodized salt by private firms and its unlimited distribution to the entire country. However, effective iodine prophylaxis including a trial of water iodization, was achieved only in a few small districts. The failure to achieve adequate prophylaxis was mainly due to the virtual unavailability of iodized salt in most local stores, because of difficulties in distribution and lack of demand.

Conclusions and recommendations
  On the basis of the above considerations the following conclusions can be drawn: (a) iodine deficiency is the cause of endemic goitre and several other disorders; (b) iodine prophylaxis with iodized salt, if correctly performed,

prevents IDD; (c) moderate to severe iodine deficiency and endemic goitre are present in several areas of Italy, and most if not all the country should be considered at least subendemic; (d) a valid iodine prophylaxis programme has not yet started in Italy.

The need for the urgent implementation of suitable legislative measures for effective iodine prophylaxis is widely recognized. We propose that the distribution of iodized salt in substitution for 'normal' salt should be made compulsory by law. Alternatively, we recommend that the consumption of iodized salt should be favoured by limiting the sale of 'normal' salt only to those persons specifically asking for it. In any case, the availability of iodized salt should be made mandatory in each food store, ensuring that at least 50 per cent of displayed salt is iodized, and that there should be no difference in the price between 'normal' and iodized salt.

Finally, to guarantee full success for iodine prophylaxis, the following proposals are also made: (a) a programme of health education using mass media and social marketing approaches should be instituted in all the country to teach the population the advantages of iodine prophylaxis; (b) centres for the control and monitoring of the effectiveness of iodine prophylaxis should be established in each Regional State.

The meeting of the Italian Thyroid Association held in Parma Italy, November 1987, further discussed the problem of IDD control in Italy. As already mentioned, iodized salt is covered by legislation but is of poor quality and distribution is very limited. As a result, at the meeting, an announcement was made that the concentration of iodide had just been increased by the Minister of Health from 15–20 mg KI per kilo to 20–30 mg. The alternative provision of the more stable iodate is also now permitted. A free 1-minute spot on national TV had also been offered by the Minister. The representatives of the salt industry from both the government sector and the private sector indicated they would be willing to provide iodized salt at the iodine concentration required. The consumer representatives indicated their appreciation of their role in advocacy of iodized salt. An officer of the Nutrition and Commerce Department of Tuscany described the development of a regional education programme in collaboration with the consumer group along the lines of the social process model (Chapter 8).

A pilot study in one village in Tuscany by Dr G.F. Fenzi and Professor A. Pinchera and colleagues at the University of Pisa (1986) had found goitre present in 56 per cent of schoolchildren and 68 per cent of adults. The iodine intake was low (mean urinary iodine excretion 48.2 μg/g creatinine). Iodine prophylaxis was started on a voluntary basis with iodized salt (20 mg KI per kilo). After three years goitre prevalence was found to be reduced in schoolchildren who had used the iodized salt. No difference in goitre prevalence was found in the adult population.

It seems most feasible for the initial development in Italy to be at regional level. Certain regions such as Tuscany would then provide evidence of the benefits of an IDD control programme which would lead to other regions following and eventually to a national consensus.

Summary and conclusions on IDD in Europe

1. There is evidence of serious iodine deficiency of national significance in the Federal Republic of Germany (FRG), the German Democratic Republic (GDR), Italy, Spain, Portugal, Rumania, Greece, and Turkey. None of these countries has a national iodized salt programme. There is evidence of a moderate to severe grade of IDD in all these countries.

    In Austria, Hungary, Poland, and Yugoslavia there are substantial areas with high goitre prevalence in spite of an iodized salt programme. This is due to inadequate KI content (10 mg per kilo). Increase to 20 mg KI per kilo is required.

    These countries compare unfavourably with the complete control of IDD that has been achieved by the Scandinavian countries.

2. There is clearly a need for effective national IDD control programmes in the FRG. GDR, Italy, Spain, Portugal, Rumania, Greece, and Turkey. These programmes are the responsibility of national governments. They will not succeed without the full political support of the ministers of health with appropriate cooperation from other relevant departments (education, media, and industry).

3. These programmes require an educational component in view of the sensitivity of the social issue of food additives. This is despite the fact that iodine is an essential element and therefore an essential dietary ingredient at a level of 100–200 μg per day to maintain a normal output of thyroid hormones.

4. Various technologies are available apart from iodized salt (iodized water, milk, and bread). The use of iodized oil by mouth

or injection should be considered as an alternative as it can be administered to selected groups (children and women of child bearing age) through the health care system without the need for legislation.

5. There is a need for continuous monitoring of iodine nutrition and the prevalence of IDD in schoolchildren at national and regional level in those countries with a continuing IDD problem. Suitable laboratories are required for the determination of urine iodine.

The maintenance of an adequate level of iodization of salt also requires continuous monitoring of production, distribution, and consumption.

Particular attention should be given to newborns by determination of urinary iodine levels. Checks on neonatal T_4 levels for transient hypothyroidism may also be informative.

Bibliography

Bauch, K., *et al.* (1986). Thyroid status during pregnancy and post partum in regions of iodine deficiency and endemic goitre. *Endocrinologia Experimentalis* **20**, 67-77.

Delange, F., *et al.* (1986). Regional variations of iodine nutrition and thyroid function during the neonatal period in Europe. *Biology of the Neonate* **49**, 322-30.

Fenzi, G.F., Aghini-Lombardi, F., Giusti, L.F., Marcocci, C., and Pinchera, A. (1986). Epidemiological studies on endemic goitre and IDD in Tuscany, Italy. *IDD Newsletter* **2** (4), 8-10.

Pinchera, A., *et al.* (1986). Report on current initiatives for the control of IDD in Italy. *IDD Newsletter* **2** (4) 6-7.

Scriba, P.C., *et al.* (1985). Goitre and iodine deficiency in Europe. *Lancet* **1**, 1289-93.

Further Reading

Hetzel, B.S., Dunn, J.T., and Stanbury, J.B. (eds.) (1987). *The prevention and control of iodine deficiency disorders*. Elsevier, Amsterdam.

11

Latin America

Iodine deficiency disorders occur widely throughout Central and South America. However, the most severe IDD occurs in the Andean region extending the whole length of South America from Colombia through Ecuador, Peru, and Bolivia to Argentina and Chile. Of these the most severely affected are Ecuador, Peru, and Bolivia.

The terrain most affected is that of the Andean Sierra at an altitude of 3000–4000 metres where a population of some 10 000 000 live in a subsistence agriculture system in several countries. There is good evidence of the occurrence of IDD before the Spaniards came. However, it has been pointed out by Fierro-Benitez (1980) that 'the political system of the Incan Empire based on the ideal of the common good ensured that there was a well organized distribution of iodine-rich salt which was produced in the present Ecuadorean

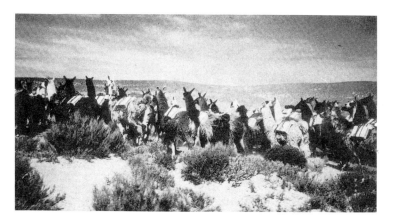

Fig. 11.1. Llama train carrying salt from Salar de Uyuni in Bolivia. Extensive salt deposits and primitive transport complicate the iodization of salt. (From *IDD Newsletter* Vol. 3, No. 1, February 1987, with permission.)

Village of Solinas and was carried as far as Cuzco, the Incan capital, because of its known curative properties for goitre'.

Fierro-Benitez goes on to point out that 'The invasion of the Europeans led to the break-up of the Incan Empire based on an agrarian system, which led to dispersal into small communities and economic chaos. There was an 'explosion' of goitre and cretinism among the rural population.'

This sequence of events prepared the way for the widespread occurrence of IDD observed in the 20th century from the 1930s onwards. The rural peasants remained isolated from the main stream of political and social change. Fierro-Benitez points out that the continued instability of many Latin American countries militates against significant public health action.

It is of interest to recall (as mentioned in Chapter 1) that the iodization of salt as a means of preventing goitre was first suggested by Boussingault in 1831. Boussingault lived for many years in Colombia where he learned from the local Indians of the beneficial effects of salt obtained from the abandoned mine in Guaca in the Department of Antioguia. He analysed the salt and found that it contained large quantities of iodine.

The modern scientific study of goitre and cretinism has been led by observations in Latin America. These began with the visit to Mendoza, Argentina in 1951 by Dr John Stanbury and his team from the Thyroid Clinic of the Massachusetts General Hospital. This team was the first to use radio-iodine in the field and so carry out dynamic studies of iodine metabolism. These studies established the association of iodine deficiency with endemic goitre and endemic cretinism. They have been the model for many other similar studies in the remote parts of the world where IDD is found. It is this body of global data which now provides the foundation for public health programmes. Stanbury also initiated a notable series of scientific meetings on endemic goitre with the support of PAHO—in Caracas, Venezuela (1963), Cuernavaca, Mexico (1965), and Puebla, Mexico (1968). These have been particularly concerned with the pathophysiology of goitre and its prevention. The proceedings of the last meeting were published (1969).

The fourth meeting, in Gauruja, Brazil (1973), took up the question of cretinism and the other complications of iodine deficiency. It provided an important coverage of public health aspects. An important series of recommendations on definitions of goitre and cretinism, research strategies, and iodine prophylaxis, led the way to global approaches to IDD control (Dunn and Medeiros-Neto 1974).

The fifth meeting was convened by PAHO in Lima in November 1983 to review the current status of the control of endemic goitre, cretinism, and iodine deficiency. This meeting was attended by public health professionals from individual countries and international agencies including PAHO and UNICEF, as well as endocrinologists and planners. Special attention was given to the public health aspects in Latin America, but some coverage of the problem in Asia and Africa was also included. The conference noted the delay in the application of the scientific knowledge. The need for the translation of knowledge into action was seen as urgent. This lag in the development of significant public health interventions had occurred in spite of the passage by 1973 of suitable salt iodization legislation in 17 of 18 Central and South American countries in which iodine deficiency was recognized as a public health problem.

At the 1973 meeting, Schaefer (1974) had provided a useful review of the factors involved in this delay based on the results of a questionnaire sent to the ministries of health of the individual countries. The factors reported by Schaefer included the following:

(1) The people, and especially the politicians, are unaware of the severity and magnitude of the problem and its detrimental effects on health, especially in regard to the sequelae of cretinism, deaf-mutism, and other serious neurological defects. There has been a failure to inform the public about the seriousness of the problem and its simple solution.

(2) The most seriously affected populations usually live in isolated rural areas where the level of social and economic development is very low. This means that the problem has little if any political impact.

(3) The traditional system of salt production is not conducive to control, and the governments fail to provide incentives to the small salt producer.

(4) The national salt commissions and government health departments fail to enforce the law. The usual pleas cite the lack of public health personnel for control activities and 'overwork'. Most of the control procedures do not require technical personnel trained in public health.

(5) There is a lack of cooperation between the industry and the public health officials or government enforcing agencies.

(6) The price of iodized salt has increased by approximately 40–60 per cent in some countries. With the simplified enrichment plants, the extra cost per kilo of iodized salt has been and still is infinitesimal.

(7) The large number of salt-producing plants makes control difficult. This basically affects only Brazil, with nearly 190 plants, and El Salvador, with 37.

The present status of IDD control in Latin America

As already mentioned, the status of IDD in Latin America was extensively reviewed at the Lima meeting and more recently at the ICCIDD Inaugural Meeting at Kathmandu in March 1986 (Pretell and Dunn 1987). Available data on goitre prevalence in Latin America are summarized in Table 11.1 for 18 Latin American countries. These data are clearly out of date for a number of countries (Argentina, Brazil, Colombia, El Salvador, Honduras, Mexico, Panama, and Paraguay).

Considerable success in the control of goitre has been achieved in *Argentina* which has had a compulsory national programme of salt iodization since 1970. Over 99 per cent of the total population is receiving iodine prophylaxis. All salt for human and animal

Table 11.1 *Goitre prevalence in Latin America*

Country	Year	Area	Prevalence
Argentina	1967	Regional	15.6
Bolivia	1983	National	65.3
Brazil	1975	National	14.7
Chile	1982	Santiago	18.8
Colombia	1965	Caldas	1.8
Costa Rica	1979	National	3.5
Cuba	1983	Baracoa	30.3
Ecuador	1983	Sierra	36.5
El Salvador	1969	National	48.0
Guatemala	1979	National	10.6
Honduras	1968	National	17.0
Mexico	1950s	Regional	5–46
Nicaragua	1981	National	20.0
Panama	1975	National	6.0
Paraguay	1976	National	18.1
Peru	1986	Sierra/selva	42.3
Uruguay	1980	Regional	2.0
Venezuela	1981	National	21.3

From Pretell and Dunn (1987) with permission.

consumption is enriched with iodine (1/30 000) using either iodide or iodate. There is indirect evidence of an adequate iodine intake. Some more remote areas have remained goitrous and oral iodized oil has been used with success. However there is some uncertainty about the continuity of the IDD control programme because the responsibility rests with regional governments. In 1980 a national seminar held at Santa Rosa recommended the use of oral iodized oil.

In *Brazil*, laws and iodization programmes were ineffective as demonstrated by high goitre rates in schoolchildren in 1975. In 1977 a new law was passed requiring 20 mg iodate per kilo of salt. However, the salt iodine content remained low. Since 1983 iodine has been made available without charge to the salt refineries by the ministry of health. This has meant deliveries to 186 refineries with monitoring of iodine content at both production and marketing sites. In 1983 the level was low but has now increased with some evidence of reduction in goitre prevalence (Pretell and Dunn 1987).

The three most severely affected Latin American countries are Ecuador, Peru, and Bolivia which will now be considered in some detail. Reference will be made to the detailed reports on these three countries which appeared in the *IDD Newsletter* of February 1987. Dr Dunn, the Editor of the Newsletter, attended a regional IDD meeting in Sucre, Bolivia in October 1986 as an ICCIDD consultant. There were representatives from Ecuador, Peru and Bolivia, as well as PAHO and UNICEF. The reports submitted were supplemented by information from the respective Directors of the National Programmes: Dr Mauro Rivadeneira, Chief of the Goitre Programme, Ecuador; Dr Eduardo Pretell, Chief of the Office for the Control of IDD, Peru; and Dr Maria del Carmen Daroca, Chief of the Division of Nutrition, Bolivia.

Ecuador

A survey in 1983 in the Sierra, where about half the Ecuadorean population of 9 million is living, revealed an overall goitre prevalence of 36.5 per cent in schoolchildren. All ten provinces were affected ranging from 29 per cent (Canar) to 48 per cent (Tungurahua). The prevalence increased with altitude. Urinary iodine levels were low.

This high prevalence was evident in spite of legislation requiring iodization of all salt for human consumption. There was a failure to include salt used for animals in the legislation so that a non-iodized salt was consumed in rural areas. The situation was clearly unsatisfactory.

In 1984 the ministry of health of Ecuador with external help from the Government of Belgium started a pilot programme in three central provinces: Cotopaxi, Tungurahua, and Chumborazo which include about 74 per cent of the iodine deficient population in the Sierra. Thirty to 35 per cent of the schoolchildren had goitre.

The programme provided for the introduction of a strict monitoring system for all manufacturers of iodized salt, both at the sites of production and distribution. Most of the salt (85 per cent) came from a major producer (Ecuasal) near Salinas. The price was three times that of non-iodized salt. However, aggressive marketing has increased the demand and availability of iodized salt in most rural areas as well as all urban areas.

Efforts are being made to organize small producers into cooperatives for the iodization of salt (with potassium iodide).

The monitoring indicates a good penetration of iodized salt into the Sierra villages. An assessment is being made of each new village with reference to salt consumption and the presence of mental retardation. If iodized salt is used by less than 50 per cent, and if mental retardation is present, there is a search for cretins. School surveys are carried out and the urinary excretion of iodine determined. If urinary iodide is less than 30 μg/day then an iodized oil injection is given (in the dosage recommended in Part II , Chapter 7). So far, only five village communities have required this intervention.

An education programme has been carried out in the villages and schools using slide shows to demonstrate the nature and control of IDD. This programme is being assessed with the help of a social scientist. Monitoring is carried out by determination of salt and urine iodine levels as well as by goitre prevalence.

As a result of these efforts there has been a big increase in the use of iodized salt in the Sierra. This can be attributed to aggressive marketing by private salt producers supported by the Ecuadorean National Goitre Programme and the Belgian Government.

An important development in 1987 has been the establishment of a national coordinating IDD control group. This is required to coordinate the national activities as well as the international aid programme. This includes not only the Belgian Government as a bilateral donor but also the Joint WHO/UNICEF Nutrition Support Programme (JNSP) with funding provided by the Italian Government.

Peru

A survey of schoolchildren in 1967 revealed that more than 23 per cent had goitre. Half the village communities in the Sierra and 80 per cent of those in the jungle were considered to have an IDD problem of public health significance. Legislation making iodization compulsory for all salt for human and animal consumption has been passed, but enforcement is lacking.

A new office for IDD control, the (UCIDD), Unit of Control of Iodine Deficiency Disorders was set up by the Ministry of Health in 1983. The Director is Dr Eduardo Pretell, a Senior Professor of Medicine in Peru who is also Regional Coordinator for the ICCIDD in Latin America.

The UCIDD initiated an up-to-date study of IDD prevalence, conducting a series of six regional courses of four days duration. Participants included health personnel, physicians, nurses, and sanitary workers. Two days were spent on IDD assessment in the field, where the trainees were shown how to assess goitre, collect salt and urine samples, and obtain information about the use of salt. The data were compiled and analysed in Lima. As of November 1986, data from 274 village communities in the Sierra and jungle (Selva) areas revealed an overall goitre prevalence of 42.3 per cent. Urinary samples were also collected and processed for iodine determinations.

Review of the salt iodization programme revealed that only 27 per cent of the iodized salt reaches the Sierra and Selva regions. The principal producer of salt is EMSAL, a government agency. The price of iodized salt is several times that of the non-iodized salt. Administration of iodized oil by injection has been undertaken as an emergency measure following this assessment in view of the delays in distribution of iodized salt. Some half million injections have been given since December 1986.

The IDD problem is being publicized in various ways—by the course trainees, and through the schools when surveys are carried out. IDD education is now being provided through the primary, secondary, and technical schools and the universities. EMSAL has been an important agent in this dissemination process.

The IDD control strategies being followed in Peru include all the elements in the social process model (Chapter 8). Assessment of IDD prevalence, education of the public and the politicians, planning, and then implementation, are the basic requirements for a successful programme. The initial strong support of the Government of Peru in setting up UCIDD was followed by international aid from the WHO/UNICEF Joint Nutrition Support Program (JNSP) with funds provided by the Italian Government.

Bolivia

Bolivia is a landlocked country divided into highlands, valleys, and lowland plains. The soils of all three regions are deficient in iodine. Sixty per cent of the population lives in the highlands with a median altitude of 3900 metres, a cold climate, and limited farming. The valleys (1500–2900 metres) extend from the highlands to the lowland plains in the east. The lowland plains have a sandy soil that is often flooded during the rainy seasons—characteristics associated with iodine deficiency.

The Quechua word for goitre is 'coto', and a number of place names in Bolivia are derived from 'coto' such as Cotoca, Calacoto, and Cotagaita. The concern about the problem dates from colonial days when Viceroy Francisco de Toledo sent a commission from Charea (now Sucre) to investigate the high prevalence of goitre.

Extensive national surveys in 1981 and 1983 showed a high prevalence of goitre (65.3 per cent). Data in 1985 confirmed this high prevalence (69.4 per cent) ranging from 53.4 per cent in La Paz (the capital) to 77.2 per cent in Chuquisaca. Cretinism is also prevalent.

The cretins were well known in the colonial period. The Quechua word 'opa' (meaning dumb) as well as 'pisichura' or 'pisiocko' (small heart) are commonly used to describe them in the rural areas. The cretins are used mainly as shepherds or household help and usually receive no pay. In one series of 95 cretins examined in Lavejaca, 75 per cent were neurological and 25 per cent myxoedematous. Severe iodine deficiency has been documented with very low levels of urinary iodine excretion (12–14 μg iodine per g creatinine) in schoolchildren in the village of Tiquipaya near Cochabamba. High levels of urinary calcium excretion have also been found which may indicate a role for a high calcium intake in the occurrence of goitre. A high consumption of cassava in the plains and valleys may also play a role.

Sporadic attempts have been made to introduce iodized salt into Bolivia over several decades with iodization plants established in Tarja, La Paz, and Cochabamba. However, significant problems and a very high price for the iodized salt relative to non-iodized salt meant that little progress was made.

In 1968 it was decreed that all salt for human and animal consumption should be iodized (with potassium iodate at a level 50 mg/kilo). Regulations for quality control were promulgated in 1982. Additional regulations have been introduced at municipal level which have sometimes been more effective than the national law, particularly in educating local communities about IDD and its correction.

The 1983 national programme called Pronalcobo (National Programme for Goitre Control) is under the direction of the Division of Nutrition of the Ministry of Health, which maintains close contacts with other ministries and interested parties. There are subsections for epidemiology, salt iodization, education, and administration. There are regional zones centred on La Paz and Sucre with regional offices for surveillance and local offices in contact with schools, health establishments, and the community.

The major salt deposits are in the Alteplasis, including the vast Salar de Uyuni (Fig. 11.1) and the Salar Coipasa. Until 1982, iodized salt was available only from Quimbabol, a large modern plant at Uyuni under the auspices of the national government. There are also small producers with a product of doubtful quality. These small producers feel threatened by the legislation requiring iodization because they lack the resources to do it. Bolivia has a strong tradition of cooperatives so PRONALCOBO has begun developing cooperatives of small salt producers to process iodized salt under the commercial name of ENCOSAL. The cooperatives aim to give financial and technical support and to assist with transport to markets. There is an assurance of 100 per cent sales to decrease costs and avoid monopolies and a special effort is being made to cover rural areas with the highest prevalence of IDD. Profits from the operation are to be returned to Pronalcobo for the IDD control programme. There are now seven cooperatives established or planned involving 783 separate producers.

The development of cooperatives has greatly altered the marketing of iodized salt in Bolivia. In the period from 1984 to

1985, there were only two major producers of iodized salt, producing 1860 metric tons. With the entrance of the cooperatives, the annual production increased to 5910 tonnes in the period 1985–86, and 9086 in 1986–87. Encosal's share of the market was 21 per cent in 1985–86 and 36 per cent in 1986–87. There are marked differences in the distribution of production costs for the cooperatives when compared with those for Quimbabol. For the cooperatives, 69 per cent of the costs is for the raw salt as opposed to 4 per cent for Quimbabol; however, cost of transportation, depreciation, and administration are much less for Encosal. This has allowed the cooperatives to sell iodized salt at 59 per cent of the price of the Quimbabol product. The lower costs of Encosal have led large private producers such as Quimbabol to decrease their prices by 50 per cent to remain competitive. Thus, more iodized salt is now available in Bolivia, at a price lower than one-half of its previous cost.

Current estimates are that 61 per cent of the total population consumed iodized salt in 1986, compared to 40 per cent in 1985 and 13 per cent in 1984. Many rural people buy salt in large 6 kg blocks, which they share with their animals. Pronalcobo has developed a plan for iodization of these large salt blocks. Current data suggest that these blocks remain satisfactorily iodized for four months. Iodization levels are checked at the plants and have, in general, been satisfactory for the products from the cooperatives.

The price to the consumer of iodized salt is about twice that of the available uniodized product, varying with the location and its distance from the site of production. For example, in La Paz, 5 kg of block salt was found to cost US $0.60, granular salt, US $0.10 per kg, refined uniodized salt US $0.16/kg, while the iodized salt of Encosal costs US $0.23/kg. However, Encosal is rapidly expanding its market, particularly in the cities, and the price differential is expected to decrease.

Summary and conclusions on IDD in Latin America

1. Since 1983 there has been a notable increase in the impact of IDD control programmes in Ecuador, Peru, and Bolivia, the three countries with the most severe IDD.

These programs have been initiated by the respective national governments with the assistance of international aid agencies—both bilateral (Belgium in the case of Ecuador) and multilateral (the JNSP programme of WHO and UNICEF with funds provided by the Italian Government to Ecuador, Peru and Bolivia.

2. The authority for the development of the programme rests with the national governments, usually with a specialized department of the ministry of health, but includes intersectoral arrangements with the other departments as in Bolivia and Peru, or with a national IDD control group as in Ecuador.

    However, there is a need for a national IDD control commission with full political authority and the responsibility for the development of the national programmes.

3. These national programmes have been initiated following IDD situational analysis by surveys for goitre prevalence, measure of urine iodine excretion, and study of the ecology of salt production with a view to the feasibility of salt iodization.

4. The development of the programmes has included all the objectives or elements of the social process model for IDD control which was described in Chapter 8. These include:

    (a) *education and communication* directed to the general public, to the politicians, to the schools, and to the health service personnel. This has been most clearly demonstrated in Bolivia.

    (b) *planning and management* involving the necessary logistics, training, supply of iodized salt, oil, or other iodine technology and the establishment of an intersectoral group evident in all three countries.

    (c) *political decision* to allocate the necessary resources. This depends on an awareness of the IDD problem by politicians and the public.

    (d) *implementation*, which has included both an emergency phase, usually with iodized oil for regions with severe IDD (as in Peru and Bolivia), and a maintenance phase with iodized salt (Ecuador, Peru, Bolivia).

    (e) *evaluation* by assessment of goitre prevalence, urine iodine excretion, serum thyroxine, and salt iodine levels. This has led to the recognition of the inadequacies of the salt iodization programme and the development of new plans to overcome the obstacles either by upgrading the salt programme as in Ecuador or by the use of iodized oil as in Peru and Bolivia.

Bibliography

Dunn, J.T. and Medeiros-Neto, G. (eds.). (1974). *Endemic goiter and cretinism; continuing threats to world health.* Scientific Publication No. 292. PAHO, Washington.

Dunn, J.T., Pretell, E.A., Daza, C.H., and Viteri, F.E. (eds.) (1986). *Towards the eradication of endemic goiter, cretinism and iodine deficiency.* Scientific Publication No. 502, PAHO, Washington.

Fierro-Benitez, R. (1980). Political, cultural and legal issues in developing prophylactic programs: A perspective from Ecuador. In *Endemic goiter and endemic cretinism: iodine nutrition in health and disease* (eds. J.B. Stanbury and B.S. Hetzel) pp. 491–95. Wiley, New York.

Pretell, E.A. and Dunn, J.T. (1987). Iodine deficiency disorders in the Americas. In *The prevention and control of iodine deficiency disorders* (eds. B.S. Hetzel, J.T. Dunn, and J.B. Stanbury, pp. 237–48. Elsevier, Amsterdam.

Schaefer, A.E. (1974). Status of salt iodization in PAHO member countries. In *Endemic goiter and cretinism: continuing threats to world health* (eds. J.T. Dunn and G.A. Medeiros-Neto). Publication No. 292, p. 272. PAHO, Washington.

Stanbury, J.B., (ed.). (1969). *Endemic goitre.* Scientific Publication No. 193. PAHO, Washington.

Further Reading

Dunn, J.T., Pretell, E.A., Daza, C.H., and Viteri, F.E. (eds.). (1986). *Towards the eradication of endemic goitre, cretinism, and iodine deficiency.* Scientific Publication No. 502. PAHO, Washington.

Stanbury, J.B. and Hetzel, B.S. (eds.) (1980). *Endemic goiter and endemic cretinism: iodine nutrition in health and disease.* Wiley, New York.

12

Asia

The largest populations suffering from iodine deficiency are found in Asia in significant proportions of three of the world's most populous countries—China, India, and Indonesia—as well as in a number of other countries. As expected, the reason for the deficiency is the low iodine content of the soil in which the staple food crops are grown. These are mountainous areas, as in the region of the Himalayas and the many mountain ranges of China. But they also include river valleys subject to periodic flooding as in the Ganges valley of India and Bangladesh, the Songkla valley of Northern China, and the Irawaddy valley of Burma. These river valleys are fertile and hence large populations live in them and are usually totally dependent on the local food crops, which are inevitably iodine deficient whatever their nature. China provides a vivid example: iodine deficiency is widely prevalent whether the main staple is wheat as in the North, corn as in the West, or rice as in the South.

My own experience of the problem of IDD in the field has been in Asia following on our earlier work in New Guinea over the period 1964–1972. This experience began in Indonesia in 1976 when I first visited Central Java at the invitation of Dr. R. Djokomoeljanto, Professor of Medicine of the Faculty of Medicine, Diponegoro University in Semarang. Semarang is the provincial capital of the province of Central Java which contains 27 million people. I was appointed as an international consultant to the Indonesia program in 1978 and have visited Indonesia on a number of occasions over the past ten years.

I visited China first in 1981 as a member of a Water Resources Delegation of the Australian Academy of Science. On arrival in Beijing I received a letter of invitation from Professor H.I. Chu to visit Tianjin Medical College of which he was the founding President. Professor Chu (who died at the end of 1984) was the pioneer in the use of iodized salt in China in 1961–62 but the program had disintegrated under the impact of the Cultural Revolution over the ten-year period 1966–1976. Professor Chu was well aware of our work in Papua New Guinea through our publications and asked me to lecture on it in Tianjin. On my first visit to Tianjin I was met at the railway station with much enthusiasm by Professor T. Ma and colleagues. Their account of the massive problem of IDD in China made a vivid impression on me. For many years they had been isolated from Western scientist colleagues, but they knew of our work on the sheep model, from the careful and comprehensive reading of the published scientific literature which is so characteristic of our Chinese colleagues. This first mutually enthusiastic contact with Chinese colleagues rapidly led to discussion of future collaboration on scientific studies involving animal models.

In 1982, Professor Ma spent three months at the CSIRO Division of Human Nutrition working on the sheep model and the micro-determination of iodine in our laboratories.

It has been my privilege during three separate visits (1981, 1982, and 1984) to see and discuss the IDD problem of China in a number of provinces with the help of Professor Ma and Professor Chu. These provinces include Sinjiang and Chinghai (West China), Heilongjiang (North-east China), Guizhou (South China), and Hebei and Henan (Central China). Particular attention has been focused on the problem of endemic cretinism, as discussed in Chapter 3. These visits led to the Australia–China Technical Agreement for the Control of IDD in China (1986–1991).

Lastly, I have been involved in the Himalayan Region (India, Nepal and Bhutan) through a series of visits since 1983. In 1983 I gave a lecture on iodine-deficiency disorders at the Indian Council of Medical Research in New Delhi. Later that year I was Chairman of a Symposium on Iodine Deficiency in Asia at the Fourth Asian Congress of Nutrition in Bangkok. This was the first occasion in which the full dimension of the IDD problem in Asia had been presented to an International Nutrition Conference.

This chapter will concentrate on three different regions or countries.

(1) *The Himalayan and Sub-Himalayan Region*—India, Nepal, Bhutan, Burma, Bangladesh, and Pakistan, where the people live in mountains, hills, or flooded river valleys;

(2) *Indonesia*—the Archipelago of 13 000 islands where 163 million

people live on the coast, or inland in hilly areas often associated with volcanoes;

(3) *The People's Republic of China (PRC)*—the most populous nation on earth where more than 1 billion (1 050 000 000) live in a predominantly mountainous environment.

In Chapter 6, estimates were presented of the prevalence of IDD for the different countries of the WHO South-east Asian Region. These were derived using a mathematical model developed by the epidemiologist Eric Dulberg based on extensive survey data on the prevalence of goitre and cretinism in these countries. The estimates are summarized in Tables 6.4, 6.5, and 6.6. The massive impact of iodine deficiency on these countries is clearly demonstrated. Overall there are nearly 250 million with goitre in a total population of over 1 billion people in the eight countries of the South-east Asian Region.

This region does not include the massive population of China which is in the Western Pacific Region of the WHO along with Vietnam, Laos, Kampuchea, Malaysia, the Philippines, and Papua New Guinea. All six of these smaller countries have significant IDD problems related predominantly to mountainous areas.

Approximately one third of the population (300 million) of the People's Republic of China live in an iodine deficient environment. This huge population represents a big challenge to effective prevention and control. As we shall see, the Chinese have made remarkable progress even though they have only been effectively engaged since 1978 after the passing of the Cultural Revolution following Chairman Mao's death in 1976.

We shall now consider in detail the current control of IDD, evidence of success and failure, and the prospects of effective control in the next 5–10 years. It could be said that effective global control of IDD now depends on control in the Asian and African countries.

The Himalayan and Sub-Himalyan Region

India has been a major site of activity in the definition and control of IDD since the early 1900s when McCarrison described goitre and cretinism in the Western Himalayas—the Karokoram Range in what is now Pakistan (see Chapter 2). The subsequent work of Professor V. Ramalingaswami and colleagues in defining the role of iodine deficiency, and the demonstration of the effectiveness of iodized and iodated salt in the Kangra Valley Region of Himachal Pradesh have provided the basis for the control programme in India and in the surrounding countries of the Himalayan and Sub-Himalayan Region (see Chapter 7).

India

A high prevalence of goitre exists in the Himalayan–Sub Himalayan belt extending from Jammu and Kashmir in the west to the Naga Hills in the east. This belt extends at least 500 kilometres south of the Himalayas into the flat Sub-Himalayan Terai (plains) of the Ganges Valley. There are at least 150 million people living in this area, which includes 15 States (Jammu and Kashmir, Himachal Pradesh, Punjab, Hanyara, Uttar Pradesh, Bihar, West Bengal, Sikkim, Assam, Mizoram, Meghalaya, Tripura, Manupur, Nagaland, and Aranachal Pradesh). Of these, 55 million people are estimated to have goitre.

Goitre also exists in many other areas of India. Surveys over the past 10 years reveal that 16 of India's 22 States, and 4 of the Union Territories have an IDD problem (Fig. 12.1). A conservative estimate using the epidemiological model described in Chapter 6 suggests that of the current population of 746 million, 150 million are at risk of IDD, 54 million actually have goitre, 2.2 million suffer from cretinism, and an estimated 6.6 million are affected by milder neurological defects attributable to iodine deficiency (Tables 6.4, 6.5, 6.6).

The National Goitre Control Programme (NGCP) of India began in 1955. It aimed to survey the problem, produce and supply iodized salt, and then resurvey after 5 years to assess the impact of the iodized salt. An iodization plant was purchased in 1956 from England and installed at one of the major salt production sites, the Sambhar Lake (Rajasthan). It had a capacity of 5 tons per day—the iodized salt being produced by dry-mixing of potassium iodide (KI) and later potassium iodate (K103) using calcium carbonate as a blender. The level was 15 ppm of iodine using salt made from subsoil brine.

Over the period 1960–65 an extensive trial was carried out by Ramalingaswami's group in the Kangra Valley district (population 100 000) in Himachal Pradesh. This revealed successful control of goitre after 3 and 5 years. The detailed data have already been

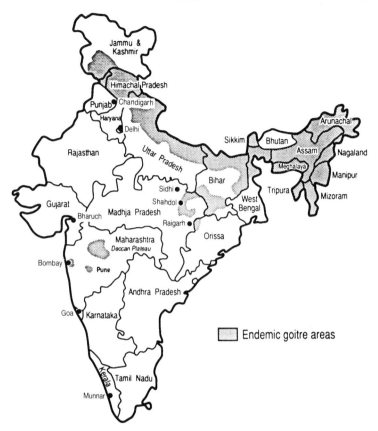

Fig. 12.1. Distribution of endemic goitre in India. (Redrawn from WHO/SEARO 1985, with permission.)

discussed (Chapter 7, Table 7.1). The superiority of iodate over iodide in the moist tropical conditions was also clearly shown.

This successful pilot study led to a large iodated salt programme being launched by the government of India with the help of UNICEF. Spray type plants were installed in Sambhar Lake (Rajasthan), Kharaghoda (Gujarat) and Howrah (Calcutta). The total installed capacity was 385 000 tonnes per year. However, the actual annual production was only about 200 000 tonnes, of which 100 000 tonnes were needed to supply Nepal. This left only 100 000 tonnes to meet an annual requirement of 400 000 tonnes for India.

In 1983, the Nutrition Foundation of India carried out an independent investigation which revealed many problems. The report suggested better intersectoral coordination and the need for better management, as well as heightened awareness by the population of the IDD problem. In response, the Government of India appointed a Working Group on Salt Technology under the Chairmanship of the Salt Commissioner Mr P. Subramanian. This Group noted the seriousness of the problem and finally recommended universal iodization of salt for the prevention and control of IDD to be achieved by 1990. The reasons for making this recommendation were:

(1) the difficulty of keeping out non-iodized salt from endemic areas;
(2) the prevalence of goitre and IDD throughout the country and the recognition that it was a national health problem;
(3) the lack of ill effects of iodized salt in normal healthy individuals.

The Government accepted these recommendations and made the historic decision to iodize all edible salt in a phased manner by 1992.

The programme has been included in the 7th Five Year Plan (1985–90) of the Government of India with an outlay of RS 210 million. The 20-Point Programme announced in 1986 aims to iodize about 52 million tons of salt by 1992. This is a very large programme, with great problems of production and distribution in view of the difficulties already encountered.

There are about 10 000 salt producers throughout India producing 9 million tons of salt by solar evaporation in salt pans. Of these, 6221 have units with an area above 100 acres the others are below 100 acres including 1831 who are small manufacturers working without official permission. The high endemic areas along the Himalayan and Sub-Himalayan belt require rail or sea transportation over 100–2000 kilometres from the salt works in Gujarat, Rajasthan, and Tamil Nadu. This is shown in figure 12.2.

Both spray and submersion processes are used for salt iodization in India. The spray process has been standardized by UNICEF in a plant with a capacity of 5 tons per hour. The machinery is made locally at a cost of 300 000 rupees. The salt is submerged in a solution of potassium iodate for about five minutes and the solution is drained out. The salt is heaped and dried overnight. This process

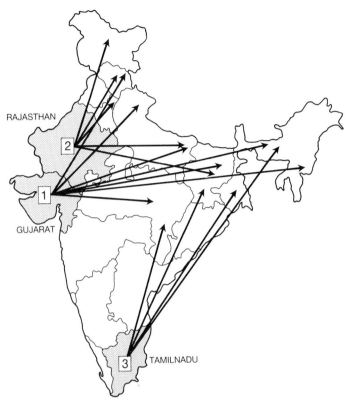

Fig. 12.2. Map of India showing movement required for the transport of iodized salt from the main salt production centres (Rajasthan, Gujarat, and Tamilnadu) to the areas with iodine deficiency. (From Subramanian 1987, with permission.)

is suitable for small units and has a standard annual capacity of 6000 tons. The level of iodization is 25–35 mg/kilo of K103 at the production site to provide 15 mg/kilo at the site of consumption. It is packed in specified bags of 75 kg capacity and repacked at retail level in polythene packets of 0.1 and 1.0 kg. Each unit has a quality control laboratory with analyses of iodine being carried out at regular intervals each day. Regular samples are drawn for checking by the salt department of the government.

The Ministry of Health and Family Welfare has charge of policy on the control of IDD. The salt department is under the Ministry of Industry and has the responsibility for monitoring production, distribution, quality control, and subsidy payments to the manufacturers of iodized salt.

Each state government has a 'goitre control cell' which periodically surveys the prevalence of goitre, and reports to the Ministry of Health and Family Welfare. The state governments are responsible for their own distribution of iodized salt either through the public distribution systems or the open market. The annual requirement of each state is calculated on the assumption that each individual requires 6 kg per year which also includes the requirement for animals.

Appropriate training programmes have begun for both operators and technicians in quality control, for the distribution of salt. State seminars are being held for professionals, and media campaigns are in progress to enhance public awareness of IDD through TV, radio, and newspapers. A particularly intensive media campaign has been launched in Uttar Pradesh.

The Salt Commissioner, Mr P. Subramanian, has pointed out that one of the greatest bottlenecks is the lack of an indigenous source of iodine. The entire requirement must be imported (mainly from Japan) before conversion to K103 with the necessity for foreign exchange. Another big problem is the fact that about 8000 small scale producers are manufacturing about 60 per cent of the edible salt; they need to be motivated with the provision of small scale units capable of iodizing 100–1000 tons of salt per year. These problems are very substantial indeed in the light of the previous difficulties India has had with the National Goitre Control Programme.

So far, iodized oil has only been used in a pilot programme involving the administration both orally and by injection to 10 000 children in the Gonda District of Uttar Pradesh. After 12 months there was a drop of about 50 per cent in the prevalence of visible goitre following both oral and injected iodized oil and a decrease from 63 per cent to 10 per cent in the prevalence of those with urinary iodine excretion of less than 50 μg per gram creatinine.

Other important developments in India include the establishment of IDD monitoring laboratories at the State level, the reference laboratory service, and the training programmes being run at both the All India Institute of Medical Sciences, New Delhi, and the

National Institute of Nutrition, Hyderabad. Reference has already been made (Table 6.3) to the neonatal screening service that is being developed by Kochupillai and colleagues at the All India Institute of Medical Sciences. Research is also under way into the local production of iodized oil and the double fortification of salt with iodine and iron in view of the massive problem of iron deficiency anaemia.

India remains the major challenge in the prevention and control of IDD in the world today. The new drive and purpose evident at government level needs to be transmitted to all levels of staff and personnel involved in a major national campaign with the personal sponsorship of political leaders at both national and state level. All of India's medical schools should be part of this effort.

Nepal

Nepal has a major IDD problem which poses special difficulties because of the mountainous terrain and problems of communication. Geographically Nepal is land-locked, sandwiched between China and India, with a population of 16 million covering an area of 141 577 km. The country can be divided into three parallel geographic regions extending from east to west. These are the Terai (the plains) covering the southern region, the hills ranging in height from 300–3000 metres, and the high mountains in the north reaching a height above 3000 metres. Approximately 60 per cent of the population live in the hilly and mountainous regions.

A survey of goitre prevalence carried out in 1965–66 on a sample of 5265 persons of 13 or more years of age from 19 villages (from all three regions) revealed 55 per cent with goitre. Subsequently in 1969, very high rates (74–100 per cent) were found in schoolchildren in Jumla (2250 m) and in Trisuli (550 m) associated with a wide distribution of cretinism and deaf mutism. Half the population was estimated to be hypothyroid by laboratory indicators (PBI and I^{131} uptake). These were confirmed in 1976 with the finding of low levels of iodine in water, soil, and food (Delange *et al.* 1981). In the Kunde region, Ibbertson's group from New Zealand carried out thyroid function studies before and after the injection of iodized oil. (Ibbertson *et al.* 1974)

The socioeconomic impact of IDD in Nepal is very great because of the severity of the living conditions which requires all villagers to 'pull their weight' in the struggle for survival. Since 1979 the problem has received considerable attention from the Ministry of Health, with surveys being carried out in 24 of Nepal's 75 districts by March 1986. Some 48 042 persons were examined as a sample for a population of 3 368 818. Goitre prevalence was found to be 53.4 per cent with a 1.09 per cent prevalence of cretinism. This varied from 83.9 per cent (goitre) and 10.6 per cent (cretinism) in the mountains compared to 29.0 per cent for goitre in the Jummla region in Bhojpur in the hills. From the data using the epidemiological model (Chapter 6) it has been estimated that in Nepal there are 526 000 cretins and 1.6 million other persons with milder neurological defects attributable to iodine deficiency (Table 6.4).

The Government of Nepal has taken two initiatives to deal with the problem. In 1973 a Goitre Control Project was set up to be responsible for the purchase and distribution of iodated salt from India, and then in 1979 the Goitre and Cretinism Eradication Project was given responsibility for a mass iodized oil injection campaign mainly in the hilly and mountainous regions. This latter measure has been successful, as indicated by a reduction of goitre and cretinism and increase in urine iodine levels.

However, the salt iodation programme has not been effective. Monitoring of iodine levels has revealed levels below the 15 ppm which had been the aim of the Indian salt producers. In 1979, of 100 samples tested from Kathmandu, Jummla, and Rasula, none were adequately iodized. In 1984, checks from 18 samples from five mountain/hill districts were also inadequate. In 1985, another check of 43 samples revealed less than 50 per cent with adequate iodation. It is clear that there are major logistic difficulties due to delays in transport, problems with packaging, storage, and delivery to the more remote areas.

Now the government of Nepal is building its own six iodation plants located at a series of border towns with support from India. The aim is to increase production of iodated salt to 150 000 tons per year. In the meantime India will continue to supply the iodated salt.

The iodized oil injection programme has been associated with the Expanded Programme of Immunization (EPI) of the Ministry of Health with technical support from WHO and logistic support from UNICEF. It began in 1980 with four target districts each year with the aim of covering 90 per cent of the total population, especially women of childbearing age and children. Up to March 1986, 2 466 571 injections had been given by specially trained vaccinators from the EPI programme, who were mostly illiterate. These covered 28 districts (20 in the mountains, 7 in the hills, and 1 in the Terai). An evaluation of this programme was carried out in 1986 by Drs N. Kochupillai, M. Karmarkar, and C.S. Pandav from the All India Institute, with UNICEF support. (Acharya 1987) The results have been briefly reviewed in Chapter 8. The data on urinary iodine indicate that the injection of 1 ml of iodized oil provided a satis-factory cover for 4 years. Iodization of the environment from urine excretion would undoubtedly have contributed to this effect.

Government teams have now begun to reinject certain remote districts first injected in the original programme. The alternative of oral administration is being considered. Laboratories for monitoring the iodine content of salt need to be established for each salt iodation plant as well as for urine iodine determinations in Kathmandu.

Bhutan

Bhutan is a tiny Buddhist kingdom which occupies a wholly mountainous terrain in the Himalayas. The total population is 1.2 million. They live in some 4500 villages in an area of 47 000 km^2 giving a density of 27 persons per km—a very low level for South-east Asia.

In 1975, a goitre prevalence survey revealed 47–68 per cent in schoolchildren and 50–53 per cent in the community. A national survey was undertaken in 1983, with WHO and UNICEF support, of 11 of Bhutan's 18 districts covering some 11 135 people. The mean prevalence of goitre was 64.5 per cent and cretinism was found in all districts, reaching 10 per cent or more of those most severely affected. A pilot neonatal screening program using cord blood on filter paper revealed 10 per cent of 650 samples testing had T_4 levels less than 4 μg/dl and TSH $> 50 \mu$ per ml.

Bhutan began a national salt iodation programme with the opening of a plant in the Indian border town of Phuntsholing in March 1985 with UNICEF support. (Dr John Dunn and I were asked to attend this function at which the iodation plans received the benefit of the full Buddhist ceremonial administered by monks.) A subsequent seminar with the district administrators revealed a keen interest in the IDD problem. The use of iodized salt for cattle was promoted. The salt was provided in polythene lined bags so that the iodine content would be maintained for the 12 months that would probably be the period before another trip could be made to the border from the upper mountain districts.

The need for urgent correction of iodine deficiency is obvious. In 1985, Dunn and I made a strong recommendation for the use of iodized oil in Bhutan until an effective iodated salt programme can be developed. Monitoring of urine iodine levels will reveal this. Iodine determinations on the salt are being carried out.

Burma

A high prevalence of goitre and cretinism in hill tribe areas of Burma was mentioned in the *Chin Hills Gazette* in 1886. A number of studies have been carried out since that time. A consolidated review by the Department of Medical Research in 1982 indicated that goitre was prevalent in nearly 50 per cent of the 314 townships in the country (Clugston *et al.* 1987). These townships occur mainly in the northern hill states—Chin, Kachin, Kayah, and Shan—where the overall goitre prevalence is 75 per cent. However, 40–50 per cent goitre prevalence is also found in the Irawaddy delta areas which are subject to repeated flooding as in the Ganges valley.

To summarize, some 36 per cent (14.5 million) of the population of Burma live in areas where goitre prevalence exceeds 10 per cent. In general, approximately 14.3 per cent (5.7 million) have goitre. Using the epidemiological model it is estimated that there are 305 000 cretins in Burma and a further 2.3 per cent of the population (914 000) with milder IDD neurological defects (Table 6.4).

In 1969 the government began an iodated salt campaign covering the Chin State with the distribution of 13 000 tons between 1969 and 1972. The goitre prevalence fell from 91 per cent to 24.7 per cent. Production continued until 1977 when it was no longer under government control—and this was followed by discontinuance of iodated salt production and then increased goitre prevalence.

In 1983, the government initiated an iodized oil campaign with UNICEF support. The target group was the 0–45 age group of both sexes but particular emphasis was given to women of childbearing age and children, as in other countries. By 1987 over 2 million injections had been given covering hyperendemic areas.

A feasibility study for long-term production, storage, marketing, and distribution of iodated salt has also begun to provide the basis for a long-term goitre control programme.

Bangladesh

The situation of Bangladesh in the Ganges Valley means that it is an iodine deficient region. Goitre is found in all 21 districts. Various surveys in the 1960s and 70s have confirmed high goitre prevalence, the two most severely affected districts being Rangpur (27.5 per cent) and Jamalpur (29.2 per cent), and some pockets with rates between 50–70 per cent.

In general, 38.1 per cent of the Bangladesh population live in areas where the goitre prevalence exceeds 10 per cent. The estimates from the epidemiological model are 354 000 cretins and more than 1 million suffering some significant mental or other neurological handicap (Table 6.4).

No national programme has yet been undertaken but several pilot projects with iodized oil and iodated salt have been undertaken and a national iodated salt programme is being planned.

One interesting possibility in Bangladesh is the trial of iodized water, which may provide the double benefit of control of water-borne infections. A pilot study has been discussed at the Institute for Diarrhoeal Disease Control at Dacca and it is hoped that it can be mounted soon.

Pakistan

The pioneering studies of McCarrison on endemic goitre and cretinism were conducted in the Chitral and Gilgit regions of what is now Northern Pakistan in the early 1900s. McCarrison, as already mentioned, first described the two types of cretinism which have been discussed in detail in Chapter 3.

Over the past 25 years, about a dozen IDD surveys have been conducted revealing one of the most severe endemias in the world. Virtually the whole population is affected in the mountainous areas with reduction to 15–40 per cent goitre rates in the hilly areas that border the plains. However the flooded plains of the Multan area are associated with goitre rates of 41 per cent in boys and 72 per cent in girls.

In the past three years serious attention has been given to the problem by the Pakistan government with help from the Aga Khan Foundation and UNICEF. An initial programme of 70 000 oral doses of iodized oil has been carried out by the Aga Khan

Foundation. This is to be followed by a further programme involving 5 million injections.

Some 600 tons of iodated salt were distributed to the Hunza people in 1978 with reduction of goitre prevalence from 60–70 per cent. There are big salt deposits available in Pakistan including a 'salt range' seen by Alexander the Great in 327 BC.

The estimated need for iodated salt for an at–risk population of 20 million is 68 000 tonnes per year, but the existing production is only 10–12 000 tonnes per year. There is therefore a great gap. However, this should be readily met because there are only a few major production sites. A government decision to establish universal salt iodation would ensure an effective national IDD control programme.

Indonesia

Though goitre was known for centuries, goitre prevalence was well documented throughout the Indonesian Archipelgo in the first half of the 20th century (Fig. 12.3). Further foci have been found in the 1980s since this map was made (WHO/SEARO 1985).

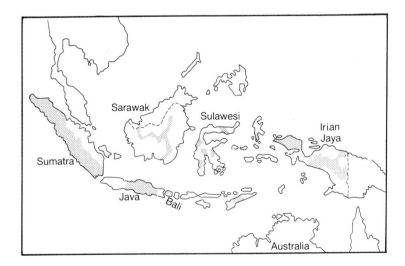

Fig. 12.3. Map of Indonesia showing shaded areas with iodine deficiency. (Redrawn from WHO/SEARO 1985, with permission.)

An extensive national survey of goitre prevalence in school-children was carried out over the period (1980–82) by I. Tarwotjo and F. Maspaitella of the Directorate of Nutrition, and by R. Djokomoeljanto of the Faculty of Medicine of Dipengoro University in Semarang (Central Java). (Djokomoeljanto *et al.* 1983) The whole country has now been mapped down to District (Kecamatan) level. Of the population of 140 million at that time, 18.5 per cent were estimated to have goitre, with the highest prevalence in Sumatra, Barat, Aceh, Jogyakarta, and Bali. From these data, using the epidemiological model, it was estimated that there were 427 000 cretins in Indonesia, with 1.3 million other persons with milder neurological defect due to iodine deficiency (Table 6.4).

Initial attempts at prophylaxis with iodized salt date from 1927 but the state monopoly of salt production was discontinued after the Second World War and iodized salt production was officially stopped in 1957.

Salt production in Indonesia comes from two major sources: the state salt factory on the island of Madura, and the so-called 'People's Salt' produced in thousands of salt pans along the Northern coast of Central Java, East Java, Bali, part of Sulawesi, Aceh, and Nusa Tenggara. This 'People's Salt' is therefore of varied origin and is in the hands of a myriad of small producers and the quality is widely variable so that it is often not suitable for iodization. Transport to different parts of the Archipelago is also a major problem.

The development of the current national programme for control of IDD dates from 1974, when both iodated salt and iodized oil injections were introduced. It is important to recognize that this major programme took its origin from the original scientific observations of Djokomoeljanto and colleagues in Central Java in collaboration with the group led by Professor A. Querido of the University of Leiden, Netherlands. These observations were concerned with both cretinism and the lesser degrees of defect demonstrable in iodine deficient areas. In-depth studies were carried out in the village of Sengi in Central Java from 1973. After the initial study of cretinism by Djokomoeljanto, which formed the basis of his thesis for the Doctorate of Medicine from Leiden University, particular attention was paid to the non-cretinous part of the population in the iodine deficient area.

The findings indicated the presence of hypothyroidism in both cretin and non-cretin groups, which indicates its more extensive prevalence than cretinism and therefore a more common cause of mental and physical impairment in the population. The more detailed studies of general intelligence and motor coordination are reported in Chapter 6.

The progress of the national programme was reviewed at a national seminar held in Semarang in December 1978. The extensive national prevalence data were presented with detailed goitre maps and progress data on the oil injection programme and the production of distribution of iodated salt reported.

It was clear in 1978 that an evaluation of the impact of the programme was required. This was subsequently carried out by Dr Eric M. Dulberg and colleagues (1983). Dulberg spent 9 months in Magelang in Central Java where he had ready access to the Sengi village community. An assessment was made of the prevalence of cretinism in all younger age groups over the period 0–16 years. Estimations of urine iodine excretion were made at the CSIRO Division of Human Nutrition in Adelaide (in 1981) and compared with the previous data obtained in Leiden in 1971. Dulberg also carried out an assessment of age of walking based on the recall of mothers for both cretins and apparently normal children.

As already noted in Chapter 8, the urine data revealed a normal range of iodine excretion indicating the effectiveness of the prophylaxis measures. The assessment of cretinism (based on the presence of mental defect and deafness, squint, or a limb weakness) revealed a prevalence of 8 per cent in children (aged 7–16) born prior to the introduction of iodine prophylactic measures in 1974. No cretin child could be found in the age group 0–7 born since iodine prophylaxis. One cretin had been born to a mother who had failed to receive an iodized oil injection.

Another striking finding was the evidence of retardation of walking age. As would be expected this was most obvious in the cretins. But it was also evident in the apparently normal children, free of other defects, born prior to iodine prophylaxis, when compared with the walking age of children born following iodized oil prophylaxis. These findings indicated a continuum of defects.

In a subsequent evaluation of the national programme, reported in Jakarta at the end of 1985, it was clear that the programme had been effective in reducing the prevalence of goitre in Sumatra,

Sulawesi, and Bali, but there was no improvement in East or Central Java. This was attributed to the difficulties in the production of iodated salt due to the myriad sources of supply, the lack of legal enforcement, and the inadequate distribution to areas of severe IDD. Only one-third of the salt supply in Java was in fact under government control and therefore readily monitored. This difficulty was regarded as almost insurmountable. It led to a recommendation for the increased availability of iodized oil, if possible in an oral preparation.

Further negotiations have taken place which have led in 1987 to the ICCIDD commissioning a feasibility study of the production of an oral iodized oil preparation by the CSIRO Division of Applied Organic Chemistry in Melbourne. This study was completed by the end of 1987 using a sample of peanut oil provided by Kimia Farma, the Indonesian Government pharmaceutical company. It is now undergoing testing in animals to be followed by clinical trials under the supervision of Djokomoeljanto in Semarang. If the preparation meets the safety requirements it will be produced by Kimia Farma and so should help greatly in the control of IDD in Java and elsewhere in Indonesia. In due course it is hoped that such a preparation will be available for African countries.

Review of the Indonesian programme indicates the importance of a series of components which together provide the basis for initiation, implementation, and evaluation. The initial assessment, planning, political decision based on an informed understanding of the scientific assessment, implementation involving logistics and training, and evaluation leading to reappraisal and a new initiative in the production of iodized oil, illustrate the social process model. The Indonesian experience is an instructive example for other countries.

People's Republic of China

The IDD group at the Tianjin Medical College, now led by Professor T. Ma following the death of Professor H.I. Chu at the end of 1984, has played a leading role since 1960 in the study and control of IDD in China. Another important group is that led by Professor Li Juanquin, formerly at Jamusi Medical College and now at Harbin Medical College. Professor Li has been responsible for the studies of the village of Jixian in Northeast China discussed in Chapter 6. His group also carried out the studies of the Jixian village diet in the rat (see Chapter 5). In 1984 Professor Li succeeded Professor Chu as the Secretary of the national leading group on IDD control in the People's Republic of China. He is now Head of the Chinese Centre for Control of Endemic Diseases at Harbin Medical College.

In a lecture given in Tokyo in 1982 at the Asia and Oceania Thyroid Association Meeting, Professor Chu discussed the status of IDD in China. According to Chu, endemic goitre and cretinism are prevalent, mostly in the mountainous regions but also in the sedimentary plains (Fig. 12.4). Reports of endemic goitre have come from all the provinces except the Shanghai Municipality. No official reports of endemic cretinism are available from Shanghai, Jiangsu, Zhejiang, Jiangsi, or Taiwan, but the presence of endemic cretinism in the last four provinces is not positively excluded. The endemic goitre rate summarized from 18 representative epidemiological surveys from different parts of the country prior to the initiation of

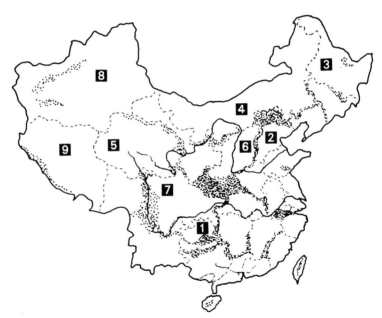

Fig. 12.4. Map of China showing IDD (dotted) areas. Some of the provinces affected include: 1. Guizhou, 2. Hebei, 3. Heilong-jiang, 4. Inner Mongolia, 5. Qinghai, 6. Shanxi, 7. Sichuan, 8. Sinjiang, 9. Tibet. (Courtesy of Professor H.I. Chu, 1984.)

iodized salt prophylaxis ran from 8.4 per cent to as high as 98 per cent in certain remote areas. The endemic cretinism rate ranged from 0.55–11.04 per cent.

Endemic goitre in China is principally due to environmental iodine deficiency, and the inhabitants in the endemic areas uniformly showed extremely low urine iodine excretion and elevated 24–hour thyroid ^{131}I uptake. So far no report has been published to demonstrate that the endemia is resistant to iodine prophylaxis. On the other hand, small isolated coastal regions where the fishermen cultivate and consume kelp and kelp-soaked salt, and certain regions where extremely iodide-rich deep well water is consumed, have been recently discovered to have iodine-excess goitre.

Since 1949 the Central Government and its Ministry of Health as well as the provincial governments concerned have legalized the supply of iodized salt to the endemic districts first in the northern part of the country, and since 1979, throughout the country except those endemic districts where iodized salt prophylaxis is impractical. The results of the wide-scale iodine prophylaxis are gratifying. Up to the end of 1979, 70 per cent of the endemic areas in Greater North China had been supplied with iodized salt, and the number of goitre patients decreased from 15 million in 1973 to 7.5 million in 1979. In 20 per cent of the endemic areas where iodized salt prophylaxis has been conscientiously practised, no new cases of endemic cretinism were discovered. Several provinces claimed to have brought the endemic disease completely under control. For instance, Shan-Xi province, once a heavy endemia, had 576 000 goitre patients in 1972, and the number of goitre patients decreased to 158 000 in 1979. Hebei province claimed to have reduced the number of goitre patients from 1 560 000 in 1972 to 390 000 in 1979.

On the subject of cretinism Professor Chu pointed out that from experience in Chenge De (Hebei province) where his group studied 80 cretins, and in Guizhou where 247 cases were studied, all were found to be predominantly of the neurological type. However, there was evidence of a number of marginal cases in the endemic areas. The evidence for this was that primary school teachers affirmed that an extraordinarily large number of so-called normal schoolchildren had failures in school records compared with children in the nonendemic areas. Furthermore, in the endemic commune of Guizhou a significant proportion of the so-called normal school-children had impaired hearing capacity indicated by audiometry and defective vestibular function. Improvement in hearing has been reported in these children following iodized salt. The results suggest effects due to juvenile hypothyroidism.

Epidemiological studies of cretinism in Guizhou province suggest recent onset.

None of the cretins was more than 20 years old. This was consistent with the evidence from old inhabitants of all three communes that goitre only became so common in the previous 20 years, and that endemic cretinism was said to be non-existent prior to 1960. Big nodular goitre was rare in older women and men which also suggested recent onset. According to the old inhabitants before 1955 all three communes were supplied with salt from the neighbouring province of Sichuan. For some reason there had been a switch to sea salt in 1955 by the three endemic communes but Qianling commune had continued with the supply of salt from Sichuan and had remained free of goitre and cretinism.

There is evidence of severe IDD in Pingliang and Heba with goitre rates of 30.4 per cent and 31.5 per cent and cretinism prevalence of 2.8 per cent and 3.1 per cent respectively, with low urinary iodine excretion. In Shilong commune there was a similar high prevalence of goitre and cretinism, but iodized salt had been introduced one year before, causing a normal urine excretion.

The major obstacle to IDD control in China is the size of the population at risk, some 300 million. The urgent need is for modern monitoring systems which will demonstrate the quality of the IDD control measures. This need is now the subject of an Australia–China Technical Agreement which provides $2.3 million over a 5-year period (1986–91). Professional training, particularly in laboratory methods, is provided as well as upgrading of equipment in laboratories to provide the necessary automation so that large numbers of samples (urine iodine and blood T_4) can be processed.

This agreement reflects the priority which IDD control is now receiving in China dating from the 11th session of the Communist Party Congress in 1978, following the Cultural Revolution (1966–76). The Cultural Revolution led to major dismantling of the IDD control programme initiated by Professor Chu. The importance of IDD control to the current one-child family policy in China is now clear to the Chinese authorities.

Recent developments in the control of IDD in China up to the end of 1986 have been summarized by Li and Wang (1987). Fifteen provinces and autonomous regions have announced that IDD has been contained based on data from monitoring and evaluation (IDD prevalence, urine and salt iodine levels).

Summary and conclusions on IDD in Asia

1. The three most populous countries of the world, China, India, and Indonesia, have severe IDD problems.
2. These large populations pose special difficulties in the supply of iodized salt, especially India and Indonesia.
3. Large programmes of iodized oil injections have been carried out to provide effective and rapid correction of severe IDD where there has been a delay in the implementation of a salt iodization programme. The countries involved include Indonesia, Nepal, and Burma. This has been assisted by support from UNICEF and the JNSP. Injections of iodized oil have proceeded without significant undesirable side effects in a total Asian population in excess of 10 million.
4. China is apparently implementing a very successful iodized salt programme since 1978 following the passing of the Cultural Revolution. This has depended on a strong political commitment.
5. Future effective programmes will require greater use of iodized oil. The recent development of oral iodized oil shows great promise.
6. The educational and communication component of the social process model (see Chapter 6) is currently illustrated in India where a major media campaign has been mounted in Uttar Pradesh.
7. Much progress has been made with IDD control in Asia in the last five years. But there is still a long way to go.

Bibliography

Acharya, S. (1987). Monitoring and evaluation of an IDD control program in Nepal. In *The prevention and control of iodine deficiency disorders* (eds. B.S. Hetzel, J.T. Dunn and J.B. Stanbury), pp. 213–18. Elsevier, Amsterdam.

Clugston, G.A., Dulberg, E., Pandav, C.S., and Tilden, R.L. (1987). Iodine deficiency disorders in South-east Asia. In *The prevention and control of iodine deficiency disorders* (eds. B.S. Hetzel, J.T. Dunn, and J.B. Stanbury) pp. 273–308. Elsevier, Amsterdam.

Chu, H.I. (See Zhu, below.)

Djokomoeljanto, R., Tarwotjo, I., and Maspaitella, F. (1983). Goiter control program in Indonesia. In: *Current problems in thyroid research*. (eds. S. Ui, K. Torizuka, S. Nagataki, and K. Miyai) pp. 403–5. Excerpta Medica, Amsterdam.

Dulberg, E.M., Widjaja, K., Djokomoeljanto, R., Hetzel, B.S., and Belmont, L. (1983). Evaluation of the iodisation program in Central Java with reference to the prevention of endemic cretinism and motor coordination defects. In *Current problems in thyroid research* (eds. S. Ui, K. Torizuka, S. Nagataki, and K. Miyai) pp. 394–7. *Excerpta Medica (Amsterdam)*.

Hou, M-T. *et al.* (1982). Epidemiologic survey of endemic goitre and cretinism in Guizhou. *Chinese Medical Journal* **95**, 7–14.

Ibbertson, H.K., Gluckman, P.D., Croxon, M.S., and Strang, L.J.W. (1974). Goitre and cretinism in the Himalayas: a reassessment. In *Endemic goiter and cretinism: continuing threats to world health* (eds. J.T. Dunn and G.A. Medeiros-Noto) pp. 129–34. Pan American Health Organization, Scientific publication 292, Washington, D.C.

Li, J.-Q, and Wang, X. (1987). Strategy for the control of IDD in China. *IDD Newsletter* **3** (4), 14–15.

Subramanian, P. (1987). Goitre and IDD control through universal salt iodation in India. *IDD Newsletter* **3** (1), 12–16.

WHO/SEARO (1985). *Iodine deficiency disorders in Southeast Asia.* SEARO Regional Health Papers No. 10, New Delhi.

Zhu, X.Y. (Chu, H.I.). (1983). The present status of endemic goitre and endemic cretinism in China, with special reference to studies in Gui-Zhou on the changes of iodine metabolism and pituitary thyroid functional status two years after iodine prophylaxis. In *Current problems in thyroid research* (eds. N. Ui, K. Torizuka, S. Nagataki, and K. Miyai) pp. 605. *Excerpta Medica (Amsterdam)*.

Further Reading

SEARO/WHO (1986). *Iodine deficiency disorders in Southeast Asia.* Delhi: WHO Regional Office for South East Asia. SEARO Regional Papers, No. 10.

13

Africa

The countries of Africa present a particularly urgent challenge for the control of IDD. More than half of the 51 countries on the continent have an IDD problem (Fig. 13.1). Many of these countries are in a considerable degree of turmoil since they became independent following the colonial era. Their governments have often been unstable, civil war has been frequent, and their agriculture is uncertain, particularly in the Sahel countries, so that famine has been a reality for millions.

It is therefore not surprising that the prevention and control of IDD has not yet received much attention from the governments of African countries. Yet it is estimated that 100–150 million of the total population of 400 million is at risk of IDD. IDD is particularly important because in virtually all these countries, 45 per cent of the population is less than 15 years of age (UNICEF estimate). When taken with women of reproductive age this makes up 70 per cent of the population in iodine deficient regions that is at risk. These countries are undergoing active development; yet iodine deficiency, as we have seen, is a formidable barrier to the attainment of self-reliance and self-determination in a competitive world.

There are a series of reports available regarding the status of IDD and IDD control in various African countries. Many of them date from the colonial era. They indicate a widespread IDD problem although it is not as extensive as in Asia, both in terms of severity and numbers affected.

In a review presented at the Inaugural Meeting of the ICCIDD in Kathmandu, Nepal, 1986, Professor O.L. Ekpechi of Nigeria, Regional ICCIDD Coordinator for Africa, pointed out the incompleteness of goitre surveys, and the discrepancies in the data (Ekpechi 1987). There are also variations in the methodology that has been adopted over so many years. Yet the data do provide an indication of the IDD prevalence in a number of countries and provide a strong indication for national programmes.

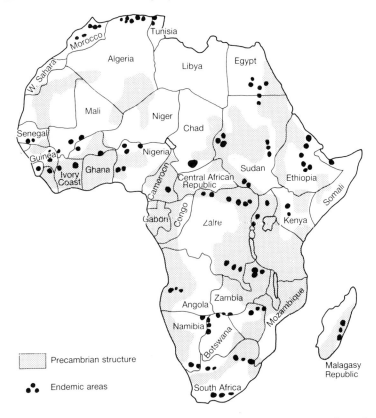

Fig. 13.1. Map showing distribution of IDD in Africa. There is general agreement on the association of Pre-Cambrian granite with areas of iodine deficiency. (From Benmiloud *et al.* 1983, with permission.)

It is of interest that the Organization of African Unity (OAU) sponsored a special seminar in 1980 calling attention to the problem and its importance for Africa.

A new IDD initiative in Africa

A new initiative for the prevention and control of IDD in Africa raises hope that indeed IDD in Africa might be brought under control to a significant degree in the next 5–10 years. The extensive research work of the Belgian group in Zaire over the preceding 20 years (Chapter 3) has been an outstanding pioneering contribution.

This initiative began in September 1985 with a consultation between the Executive Director of UNICEF, Mr James Grant, and the ICCIDD (then still in embryonic form). In a global review of the problem carried out at that time it was obvious that Africa was the continent in the greatest need, as very little was being done with national IDD control programmes.

Subsequently Ekpechi (Professor of Medicine in the University of Nigeria at Enugu, well known for his research on IDD in Nigeria over more than 20 years) and Professor Claude Thilly (Professor of Public Health at the School of Public Health in Brussels who had been actively involved in the study of IDD in Zaire) visited the Regional Director of WHO, Dr G.L. Monekosso, at the African office of WHO, Brazzaville (Republic of the Congo).

Monekosso agreed that the problem of IDD in Africa was important and one of the few problems that could readily be solved. He suggested that WHO and UNICEF might fund a Joint Regional Seminar with the ICCIDD to develop a strategy for IDD Control in Africa. WHO offered US $50 000 towards the cost. This offer was quickly taken up and plans went ahead rapidly for a Joint WHO/UNICEF/ICCIDD Regional Seminar to be held in Yaounde, Cameroon.

The ICCIDD organized a Local Coordinating Committee, which included representatives from the Ministry of Health, the Nutrition Centre, the Centre Universitaire des Sciences de la Santé (CUSS), WHO, and UNICEF. It was agreed that the Joint Seminar would be sponsored by both the ministry of health and the ministry of higher education of Cameroon.

Invitations to the seminar were then extended to the 26 African countries with an IDD problem (Fig. 13.1). It was agreed that the countries could each have two representatives—one from the ministry of health (to be funded by WHO) and one from the salt industry or with an interest in communication or health education (to be funded by UNICEF). Twenty-three countries accepted, of which 22 attended.

Joint WHO/UNICEF/ICCIDD Regional Seminar

The Joint Regional Seminar duly took place in Yaounde 23–25 March, 1987. It was attended by 34 participants from 22 African states, 17 Board members of the ICCIDD, 4 representatives of invited agencies, and 10 secretarial staff.

The Seminar found that there was sufficient data in a number of countries to justify the start of IDD control programmes. However, in many countries data were lacking, and efforts were required to secure these data so that appropriate action could be taken. The establishment of intersectoral national IDD control groups was recommended to represent the sectors of the salt industry, education and health professionals. In view of the importance to socio-economic development, the Seminar recommended that IDD control should be included in the plans for national development.

The seminar noted that methods of control would vary with each country situation. But both salt iodation and iodized oil administration for severely affected areas would have their place.

Most countries in Africa had to import salt. The principal exporters were Senegal, Egypt, Ethiopia, Kenya, Tanzania, and Namibia. The salt works in Senegal at Koalack in Sine Saloum supplied salt to about 20 countries in West and Central Africa. A regional or subregional approach to salt iodization was desirable because many African countries had relatively small populations that would not justify major iodization plants.

Nine countries presented some details of their national programmes which were at various stages of development. (Six of these will shortly be reviewed.)

The urgent need for more funding was pointed out.

In reviewing iodized oil, the Seminar noted the benefit of the mass injection programme in Zaire. However, while injections had great acceptability in some countries because of the rapid subsidence of goitre, the major AIDS problem in Central Africa indicated the desirability of avoiding injections if possible. Oral administration had been studied in Algeria and in Tanzania. The effects lasted half as long (1 ml lasts 1–2 years) as the same dose by injection (1 ml lasts 3–4 years). The advantages of the oral route were the use of less skilled staff such as community health workers and school teachers, for its administration.

An oil programme could make use of the district level primary health care structure which had been widely developed in Africa by the WHO Regional office. It would help to reinforce the value and acceptability of this district approach which covered population units of about 100 000 people.

Finally, this author proposed the creation of a task force for the control of IDD in Africa, following the example of the Child Survival Task Force that had been set up as a multiagency group in 1985 to initiate the Universal Child Immunization Programme. Such a multi-agency task force would be appropriate to the challenge presented and would lead to greater interest and financial support than would occur otherwise. Dr Bailey (WHO Regional Nutrition Adviser for Africa), Ekpechi, and this author proposed a task force with the following functions:

(1) to promote national IDD control programmes;

(2) to coordinate IDD control initiatives;

(3) to monitor progress in IDD control;

(4) to raise funds for national IDD control programmes.

To achieve this the task force would consist of an inter-agency group composed of representatives of WHO, UNICEF, ICCIDD, and interested bilaterals. This proposal had been approved by the WHO and UNICEF Regional Directors. The seminar strongly endorsed the plan.

The IDD task force

Immediately following the Joint Regional Seminar on March 26, 1987, representatives of twelve African countries (those most likely to develop national IDD control programmes) assembled with representatives from WHO and UNICEF, thirteen ICCIDD Board members, and the interested bilateral* agencies. The African countries participating were:

Cameroon, Ethiopia, Ghana, Kenya, Liberia, Mali, Nigeria, Rwanda, Senegal, Tanzania, Zaire, and Zimbabwe.

The Task Force agreed to establish three subregional groups to foster its purposes. These three groups included Eastern and Southern Africa, Central Africa, and West Africa. An ICCIDD Subregional Coordinator was appointed to each group—Ekpechi (Nigeria) for West Africa, Professor D.N. Lantum (Cameroon) for Central Africa, and Dr F.P. Kavishe (Tanzania) for Eastern and Southern Africa.

---

* Bilaterals are developed countries which provide aid directly to developing countries independently of the international agencies like WHO and UNICEF.

There was a clear need for the Subregional Coordinators to foster proposals for national programmes that would qualify for external support. They could also assist in the development of laboratory services, subregional training workshops and national seminars.

The second meeting of the IDD Task Force was held in Addis Ababa, Ethiopia, in December 1987 (Hetzel 1988). It was attended by representatives of WHO, UNICEF, Food and Agriculture Organization of the United Nations (FAO), two bilaterals (Italy and The Netherlands), and a non-government organization, Menschen für Menschen. All of these agencies were already involved in funding IDD control programmes.

The Task Force reviewed further developments in salt iodation in the light of recent reports on Kenya, Tanzania, and Malawi. In Kenya 50 per cent, and in Tanzania 25 per cent of the salt was estimated to be iodized. Both countries could export salt. In Malawi salt importers were prepared to iodate without extra charge. The possibility of universal iodation was discussed and found to be especially appropriate to the East African situation. The same could be true of West Africa where the Senegal salt mines (under French control) were so dominant; although so far iodation had been strongly resisted.

The Task Force resolved that this matter was essentially political and therefore should be brought to the attention of Heads of State in Africa in view of the recent resolution by the Organization of African Unity (OAU) on health as the foundation for development. To this end letters were written to the regional directors of WHO and UNICEF requesting them to approach heads of state for this purpose.

A level of 100 mg of iodine per kilo was recommended for salt iodation in Africa to ensure coverage for the inevitable losses during transport (up to 50 per cent) or during cooking (probably 75 per cent). Iodation at this level would undoubtedly be effective. The extra cost of a higher level of iodation was considered to be small (10 per cent) in relation to the total cost of salt production.

The Task Force spent some time discussing administrative procedures for funding national programmes. The first function was approval of the technical and administrative aspects of a proposal. There were then several alternative routes that could be used to secure funding. These included referral to UNICEF through the country programme's representative, to a bilateral agency, or to a non-governmental organization (NGO) either through WHO or UNICEF.

It was decided that it would be most appropriate for the Task Force to refer the proposal back to the ministry of health of the country with a recommendation as to the most likely source of funding. In this way the process could be expedited.

The Task Force reviewed three excellent proposals for national programmes from Tanzania, Kenya, and Zimbabwe. One feature of these proposals was their presentation as a series of separate projects, e.g., IDD prevalence surveys, communication, implementation by salt iodization and/or iodized oil, and monitoring and evaluation. Agencies could then decide which project was most appropriate for their support rather than being confronted with a decision as to whether or not they funded the whole programme.

The IDD Task Force adopted a Work Plan for 1988 and 1989 of regional and national seminars, and consultancies with multilateral and bilateral agencies and NGO's.

Recent developments in IDD control in some African countries

Six proposals for national programmes have been received by the IDD Task Force. They will now be briefly reviewed.

Zimbabwe

Zimbabwe is a landlocked country with a population of 8.6 million. It is situated on the great South African plateau—with an average altitude of 1200–1500 metres rising to above 1600 metres to the East in the Eastern Highlands.

The country became independent in 1980. A Ministry of Health with a Department of National Nutrition was formed with particular concern for IDD, malnutrition, Vitamin A deficiency, nutritional anaemia, and pellagra (Vitamin B deficiency).

Goitre has been recognized over the last 30 years. Rates of 45.8 per cent were found in 1966. A series of surveys has confirmed this and higher prevalence rates. Cretinism has been observed where goitre rates are above 30 per cent as in the Eastern Highlands. A survey in the Wedza region as recently as 1986 had confirmed similar prevalence rates to 1968—with an overall prevalence of 73 per cent in primary schoolchildren.

Studies of urinary iodine in 1985 in the Chinamora district carried out by the CSIRO Division of Human Nutrition in Adelaide revealed evidence of moderate iodine deficiency with levels of urine iodine between 25–50 μg/g creatinine. There was no evidence for the role of goitrogens. The evidence indicates the minimum population at risk to be about 3.9 million, 45.4 per cent of the total population of Zimbabwe.

IDD control has now been included in the Health-for-All Action Plan. A national plan for elimination of the IDD endemic by 1993 has now been prepared by the Deputy Director of National Nutrition, Mrs J. Butamba, and a visiting ICCIDD consultant, Dr F. Kavishe of Tanzania.

The specific objectives of the plan include:

(1) a further national survey in 1988;

(2) iodization of all salt for human consumption by 1990;

(3) administration of iodized oil orally for severe IDD endemic areas by 1990;

(4) professional and public sensitization to IDD control;

(5) strengthening existing relevant laboratories for IDD assessment for baseline and monitoring purposes;

(6) training courses for IDD control programme staff starting in 1988.

The proposed national programme has been drawn up as a series of inter-related projects designed to meet the specific objectives.

A multisectoral national council has also been recommended and this recommendation has recently been accepted by the government. Legislation is to be initiated for enforcing iodation of salt; mass communication will be supported; and mobilization of resources from both within and outside the country will be undertaken. It is important to note that all salt in Zimbabwe has to be imported.

Kenya

The Republic of Kenya extends from sea level in the east to an altitude of more than 5000 metres (Mount Kenya) in the west. The estimated population as of June 1986 was 20.1 million. The country is primarily agricultural (60 per cent of the gross domestic product). Subsistence farming is the major occupation in the Central, Myanza, Western, and Rift Valley provinces where the land is fertile with good rainfall, but iodine deficient. There is little importation of food and cassava is consumed in large quantities.

Earlier studies in schoolchildren revealed goitre prevalence between 15–72 per cent. These studies were carried out on 28 520 children aged 6–15 years in 108 schools in 14 districts from a number of provinces and were reported to the ministry of health in 1968. Endemic cretinism has not been reported in Kenya (Hanegraaf 1977).

On the basis of earlier studies of urine iodine excretion in 1974–75, approximately 12.0 million people (62.8 per cent of population) are estimated to be at risk. IDD is therefore a priority problem.

An initial attempt at salt iodation (20 mg/kilo) was made over the period 1970–72. However, no significant improvement occurred in urine iodine levels and there was no reduction in goitre prevalence. Legislation requiring salt iodation was passed in 1978 with reinforcement in 1981, but little action has been taken and iodization of salt is not being carried out in spite of the ready availability of salt at low price from within Kenya.

Interest has been rekindled following the formation of the ICCIDD. A Regional Action Plan was prepared at meetings in Gaborone (November 1986) and in Nairobi (January 1987) and subsequently endorsed by the IDD Task Force. The National Council for Control of Iodine Deficiency Disorders in Kenya was founded in November 1987.

Similar objectives were accepted as listed above for Zimbabwe. A similar national plan with a series of projects has been drawn up by Mr Tom Omondi of the ministry of health in association with ICCIDD. This proposal has now been approved by the minister of health and so can now be submitted for funding support.

Ethiopia

Ethiopia is a very poor country with chronic famine and scarce water supplies. The income of two-thirds of the population is below subsistence level. There are high rates of infant, child, and maternal mortality.

Goitre has long been recognized in Ethiopia and has been described extensively by Western travellers from the turn of the century. A series of detailed studies in various areas between 1950 and 1970 confirmed a high prevalence of goitre in the highland areas.

Between 1979 and 1981 a systematic study by the Ethiopian Nutrition Institute involved a sample of over 35 000 schoolchildren and 19 000 household members. The results indicated goitre to be widespread. Overall 25 per cent of Ethiopians (10 million people) have at least mild goitre, while 12 per cent had visible goitre. Low iodine intake rather than goitrogens was the major cause of IDD. Cretinism was seen but no systematic study has been undertaken.

The agreed main strategy for IDD control is salt iodization. Ethiopia is self-sufficient in salt, producing some 200 000 tonnes per year at two cooperatives which are directly controlled by the government. In some areas with severe IDD, iodized oil will be used.

Despite the food crisis of 1984/85, the following steps have been taken—

1. A joint IDD monitoring committee has been established (Ethiopian Nutrition Institute, Ethiopian Domestic Distribution Corporation, National Chemical Corporation, and UNICEF).

2. A local technologist has been trained in India in salt iodization techniques.

3. Laboratory equipment and two years' supply of potassium iodate have been ordered and stored.

4. Three spraying and mixing machines (6 tonne capacity) have been procured and set up at the major site of salt production (Assab).

5. In-service training of 20 existing salt works technicians on salt iodization has been provided.

The aim is for the production of over 200 000 tonnes of iodized salt per year. Quality control will be established at various distribution centres and retail sites.

The specific objective is the reduction of goitre prevalence to below 5 per cent by the year 2000 in endemic areas. Areas of severe IDD will receive special attention with iodized oil, before effective distribution of iodized salt can be achieved.

This programme has now received a grant of US $500 000 from the Menschen für Menschen Foundation (The People to People Foundation of Germany and Austria). Other funds are being sought by UNICEF.

Tanzania

In 1987 the population of Tanzania was estimated to be about 22.5 million. The country rises from sea level on the eastern coast to highlands in the south and north reaching up to 5800 metres (Mount Kilimanjaro). The Great Rift Valley with its two arms stretches through the whole country, including Lakes Tanganyika and Nasa.

Agriculture provides 60 per cent of the gross domestic product. Cassava is the main staple in the coastal zone, and increasingly on the plateau and in the highlands.

Since the early 1950s it has been clear that endemic goitre is a problem in the southern highlands. This has been confirmed by surveys in various regions of the country. A plan to iodate salt in 1973 was never implemented.

However, in 1983, the Tanzanian Food and Nutrition Centre met with the ministries of health and industry and recommended the appointment of a National Goitre Expert Committee to prepare an IDD control plan. This Committee met in 1979 and adopted a two-pronged strategy involving the use of both iodized oil (in areas with goitre prevalence of 60 per cent or more) and iodized salt for the long term. Pilot studies have demonstrated the benefits of both measures.

A national survey in primary schoolchildren was then carried out. This provided the basic data from which the various manifestations of IDD were estimated using the Dulberg model (Chapter 6). According to the model,

(1) 9.3 million people (41 per cent of the population) were estimated to be at risk of IDD;

(2) 5.0 million were suffering from endemic goitre;

(3) there were 160 000 cretins;

(4) there were 450 000 'cretinoids';

(5) 10 000 late reproductive losses occurred in 1985 or 25 deaths per 1000 live births per year.

Tanzania has been graded by Kavishe as a country with moderate IDD; 10 districts have severe IDD (10 per cent or more visible goitre rate) and 24 districts have 30 per cent or more total goitre rate.

Tanzania is determined to eliminate severe IDD before 1993. A comprehensive strategy has now been prepared. This involves a series of projects including IDD surveys, salt iodation, the development of laboratory services, iodized oil distribution, communication, training, research, consultancies, monitoring, and evaluation.

A National Council for the Control of Iodine Deficiency Disorders (NCIDD) has been established. A national seminar was held at Arusha in November 1985. Implementation of the plan began in 1986 with the administration of 500 000 iodized oil capsules (250 000 people) in the Miseya and Iringa Regions. The governments of Sweden and Holland have supported these measures.

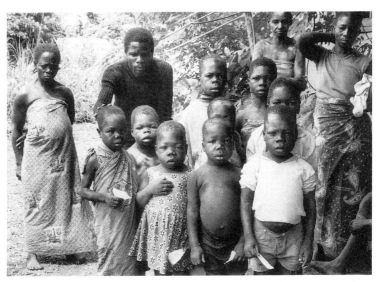

Fig. 13.2. Severe IDD in Zaire—group of myxoedematons cretins, children and adults in the age range 16–30 years. Clinically normal adults are shown at the back. (From Delange *et al.* 1981 with permission.)

Zaire

Zaire is almost landlocked with only a narrow access to the sea at the mouth of the Congo river. The estimated population for 1987 is 33 million. It is estimated that about 13 million people live in iodine deficient areas of which 5–10 million live in highly endemic areas with severe IDD (Fig. 13.2).

Salt has to be imported—mainly from Angola but also from

Tanzania. Studies of salt distribution and consumption are needed.

There is a wide prevalence of communicable diseases, especially malaria, diarrhoeal, and other parasitic diseases. The health strategy of the country centres on the development of primary health care for some 360 health zones established for the purpose, corresponding to health districts as described in the charter for health development adopted by all member States in the African region. Some 160 of these zones are now operational with health management teams and health development plans. These include maternal and child health (MCH) services and the expanded programme of immunization (EPI).

A large scale iodized oil programme has been carried out in the Equateur region with the support of the Belgian Government. This has involved over one million people.

The government has now decided that IDD is a priority second only to malaria and is committed to developing a national programme. Recently (November 1987) a multiple agency mission, including representation from UNICEF, the World Bank, and Belgium has visited the country to assist in the preparation of a national plan.

The role of cassava has been defined by the extensive research by the Belgian group of Dr Andre Ermans, Dr Francois Delange, and Dr Claude Thilly and their collaborators over more than 30 years (Ermans *et al.* 1980). The efficacy of iodized oil has been well demonstrated by the Belgian-Zairian group in the major programme in Equateur (Thilly *et al.* 1977).

It is proposed that iodized oil be administered in regions of severe IDD over the next 3–5 years. This will be followed by iodated salt distribution if it can be effectively organized. However, there is no doubt that oil will need to be continued, especially for the more remote areas.

Nigeria

Nigeria has a population of 100 million of whom 85 per cent live in rural areas. It is the tenth most populous country in the world with a growth rate of 3 per cent. It has a Federal structure with a central government under a military administration. There are 19 State governments, each administered by a military governor. Health is largely a State function.

Nigeria has an immense IDD problem. It is estimated there are 25 million people living in iodine deficient areas. So far only 37 local government areas (LGA) in 7 States have been surveyed. The situation in the remaining 267 LGAs is not known.

An expert committee on salt iodization was set up in 1974. This committee recommended that all salt consumed in the country should be iodated and that the necessary legal and trade measures be initiated.

The cost of salt iodization has been estimated to be 4 cents per capita per year (0.16 Naira). This means a cost of US $400 000 (N 16 million) per year for the population of 100 million. The total government expenditure on health is N 2.5 per person per year or N 250 million for the total population. Some help from international agencies will be available to initiate the development of salt iodization, but Nigeria itself will have to sustain the effort as soon as possible.

The development of a national IDD control programme for Nigeria is clearly a Herculean task. Previous experience with the EPI Programme provides some helpful guidelines. The EPI programme started in 1975, but after 8 years the impact on the target diseases was negligible. In its review of the shortfall in achievement UNICEF commented:

The most fundamental problem identified was that the EPI plan of operation had been developed without the involvement of state ministries of health, which are responsible for implementation and thus their commitment to a sustained long-term immunization programme had been weak.

Detailed study by a joint intersectoral committee made up by the Federal Ministry of Health, UNICEF, and WHO concluded that the following factors were responsible for the poor performance:

(1) weak management structure of the existing health services;
(2) unrealistic budgetary allocation;
(3) inadequate data base for planning and evaluation of project;
(4) ineffective health education programme;
(5) poor health information system;
(6) difficulties in reaching the remotely rural villages.

They further observed that the Community Development and Primary Health Care Workers 'seldom reach the most needy rural subsistence farmers, the illiterate mothers, etc.' Concluding, they remarked: 'Despite the huge financial investments, no significant impact on the quality of life of the vulnerable groups especially women and children in the rural areas has been made.' The EPI programme had still not been able to overcome these difficulties by 1986.

The experience indicates, as Ekpechi points out, that much more than adequate financial resources are required for successful programme implementation.

Ekpechi has now been requested by the Minister of Health of Nigeria (Dr Ransome-Kuti) to proceed with the development of a national plan for IDD control. He is beginning with the communication aspect which has previously been neglected. This has to take account of the fact that 70 per cent of the Nigerian population is out of the reach of the news media. Appropriate Federal and State committees will be formed. A national workshop is to be held in Lagos early in 1988 for the 19 State ministries of health to be followed by State workshops. The programme is planned in two phases:

1st phase 1988–1993: to cover 36.8 million people in 7 States (127 LGA) for which some reliable information is available.

2nd phase 1993–2000: to cover 63.2 million people in the remaining 12 States. These require a national IDD survey as there is no reliable baseline data.

An emergency sub-phase with iodized oil, and a long-term sub-phase with iodized salt has been adopted.

An impressive plan has been drawn up by Professor Ekpechi and his colleagues. We wish him well with a major challenge.

We hope that 1987 will be regarded as an important landmark in the control of IDD in Africa. Certainly much progress has been made through a coordinated approach.

Summary and conclusions on IDD in Africa

1. There are 100–150 million people at risk of IDD in Africa. The seriousness of the problem has been noted by the Organization for African Unity (OAU) who have recently emphasized that health is a foundation for development.
2. There is a lack of detailed survey data on IDD prevalence on which public health programmes can be based.
3. The development of national programmes for more than 30

countries requires coordinated support from international and bilateral agencies for provision of necessary expertise and funding.

4. The establishment of the IDD Task Force for Africa, on the initiative of the ICCIDD supported by WHO and UNICEF and key bilaterals, has provided regional support for the development of national programmes.

5. So far Tanzania, Kenya, Zimbabwe, and Ethiopia have completed planning with the approval of their national governments. Nigeria, Zaire, Mali, Cameroon, and Malawi are well advanced in the preparation of their national programmes.

6. The Task Force has recommended that salt iodation be carried out at a level of 100 mg per kilo. The value of the inter-dependence of the African States for the supply of iodated salt has been pointed out to the Heads of State through the OAU as a major opportunity to improve child survival and development in Africa.

7. The Task Force has also made recommendations for training seminars and workshops, the provision of laboratory services and procedures to be followed to secure funding of country programme proposals.

8. The appointment of ICCIDD Subregional Coordinators by the IDD Task Force is a further important step to provide support for the development of national programmes.

9. Africa offers a great opportunity to the world for the successful prevention and control of IDD within a decade in the face of other more difficult and long-term problems.

Bibliography

Benmiloud, M., Bachtarzi, H., and Chaouki, M.B. (1983). Public health and nutritional aspects of endemic goitre and cretinism in Africa. In *Cassava toxicity and thyroid* (eds. F. Delange and R. Ahluwalia) p. 50. Research and public health issues, IDRC, Ottawa.

Chinamora Research Team (1986). Endemic goitre in Chinamora, Zimbabwe. *Lancet*, **2**, 1198–200.

Ekpechi, O.L. (1987). Iodine deficiency disorders in Africa. In *The prevention and control of iodine deficiency disorders* (eds. B.S. Hetzel, J.T. Dunn, and J.B. Stanbury), pp. 219–36. Elsevier, Amsterdam.

Ermans, A.M., Mbulamako, N.M., Delange, F. and Ahluwalia, R. (eds.) (1980). *Role of cassava in the etiology of endemic goitre and cretinism*. IDRC, Ottawa.

Hanegraaf, T.A.C. (1977). Population based studies of endemic goitre in Kenya. *East African Medical Journal* **54**, 167–74.

Hetzel, B.S. (1988). Iodine deficiency disorders. *Lancet* **1**, 1386–7.

Thilly, C.H., Delange, F., Ramioul, L., Lagasse, R., Luvivila, K. and Ermans, A.M. (1977). Strategy of goitre and cretinism control in Central Africa. *International Journal of Epidemiology* **6**, 43.

World Health Organization. (1987). *Control of IDD in Africa.* Report of Joint WHO/UNICEF/ICCIDD Regional Seminar. Brazzaville, Congo.

Further Reading

IDD Newsletters. (1987). Focus on IDD in Africa. Vol. 3, No. 1. IDD Newsletter. (1987). IDD Task Force, Second Meeting. Vol. 3, No. 4, p. 2.

World Health Organization. (1987). *Control of IDD in Africa.* Report of Joint WHO/UNICEF/ICCIDD Regional Seminar. Brazzaville, Congo.

14

The chances of success

In the last 40 years, iodine deficiency and its effect on human potential, health, and well-being has been defined. We have seen that iodine deficiency affects many hundreds of millions of people living in iodine deficient environments. These people are to be found mostly in developing countries with large populations such as China, India, Indonesia, Bangladesh, Nigeria, and Zaire, but they are also found in Europe, particularly in the Federal Republic of Germany, the German Democratic Republic, and Italy.

The major impact of iodine deficiency on human well-being has been loss of physical and mental energy due to inadequate production of the iodine-containing thyroid hormone. This affects many people with endemic goitre apart from the gross condition of endemic cretinism.

The correction of the deficiency by use of iodated salt or iodized oil (or other means) has been shown to be followed by prevention and control of goitre and cretinism. There is also evidence of a general increase in energy and activity so that individuals and, through them, the community are able to take a new interest in life and so develop a much greater degree of self-reliance.

The cost of the available technology with iodated salt is indeed modest—3–5 cents per person per year—less than the cost of a cup of tea.

Monitoring the correction of iodine deficiency is readily achieved with measurements of the dietary iodine intake through urine iodine or by measurement of serum thyroxine (T_4) levels in the blood. These techniques have been greatly facilitated by the development of automated instruments able to process large numbers of samples.

To summarize, the iodine deficiency problem (IDD) is significant, massive populations are at risk, effective mass technology is available, and monitoring can be carried out on the required scale.

There is already a major programme in progress dedicated particularly to children in the third world. This is the Child Survival

The problem of iodine deficiency and its solution

1. Significant massive problem affecting quality of life of millions	IDD
2. Affordable mass technology for prevention and control	Iodized salt Iodized oil
3. Practical methods for assessment and monitoring	urine iodine Blood thyroid hormones
4. Public health programme for implementation	National IDD control commission
5. International resources for support	WHO UNICEF Bilateral aid ICCIDD

and Development Revolution which has been led by UNICEF, WHO and other major international agencies following consultations in 1982 (Cash *et al.* 1987).

The programme has concentrated on four simple approaches—particularly dedicated to reduction of mortality in children. They are universal immunization, oral rehydration for diarrhoea, breast feeding and better weaning, and growth monitoring of small children.

These approaches have been communicated using new social marketing techniques. There has been an emphasis on literacy with training programmes for young mothers. Radios are now available in almost every home together with one or two television sets per village. Religious and other social groupings have been involved in the mass communication effort (Cash *et al.* 1987).

Review in June 1986 revealed considerable progress—universal child immunization by 1990 has now been adopted as a goal by over 60 developing countries which include 26 with populations greater than 20 million. Vaccine use in developing countries has increased by a factor of three since 1983, use of oral rehydration salts has increased by two and a half times since 1983. It was estimated in 1985 that the deaths of more than 1 million children under the age of five years were prevented.

In his message to the Inaugural Meeting of the ICCIDD in Kathmandu, the Executive Director of UNICEF, Mr Jim Grant, indicated his belief that the control of iodine deficiency must be a priority objective within the Child Survival and Development Revolution (Grant 1987). Conclusive evidence for the importance of iodine deficiency to child survival and development is summarized in Chapter 6.

It is also clear that the prevention and control of IDD provides a major contribution to the WHO objective of Health for All by the year 2000, as pointed out in the World Health Assembly Resolution (WHO 1986).

What then are the chances of significant progress?

The effective functional unit is the National IDD Control Programme. There are three requirements for an effective national IDD control programme—

(1) *motivation of national governments* of countries with a significant IDD problem;
(2) *financial resources* mainly from the UN system, bilateral aid-giving countries, and non-government organizations until these governments can fund programmes themselves;
(3) *trained manpower* to carry out these national programmes.

1. *Motivation of national governments.* As we have seen, motivation of national governments has been occurring at an increasing pace over the past 5–10 years. China has made good progress since 1978, India since 1983, and Indonesia since 1974, and there is increasing motivation being shown in Latin America and in Africa.

Such increased motivation depends on political awareness. This is the result of advocacy by the medical and scientific community (national and international) and the international agencies (multilateral, bilateral, or NGO). There is a need for both increased national and international awareness of the great opportunity available for prevention of IDD. Suitable media coverage can assist this process, using different technologies for different situations.

2. *Financial resources* External funding is available from the UN system, bilateral aid-giving agencies, and NGOs. These agencies are becoming aware of the excellent investment in developing self-

reliance that support of national IDD control programmes provides. IDD control offers a big return. Furthermore, the costs are not overwhelming for Third World governments. This will depend on the politicians and the electorate understanding the problem, including the need for continued monitoring of the IDD control programme. Incorporation of the prevention and control of IDD within the Child Survival and Development Programme will assist financial support.

3. *Trained manpower* This includes planners, economists, nutritionists, epidemiologists, statisticians, iodine technologists, and media and communications experts. A multidisciplinary team is required that can be effectively focused by a national IDD control commission with appropriate political authority for the programme.

Some trained manpower might well be available from the Child Survival and Development Programme.

The combination of motivation, funding, and trained manpower provides the basic ingredients for a successful national IDD control programme.

These provisions all depend on an initial perception of the value both social and economic, of the prevention of IDD as a realizable goal at an affordable cost so that 'political will' can be generated.

In the end, the chances of success depend on political will which comes from people motivating their governments so that the scourge can be eliminated. There is a great opportunity—let us seize it.

References

Cash, R., Kensch, G.T., and Lamstein, J. (eds.) (1987). *Child health and survival: the UNICEF GOBI-FFF Programme*. Croom Helm.

Grant, J. (1987). Message to the Inaugural Meeting of the ICCIDD—Kathmandu, Nepal, March 25-28, 1986. In *The prevention and control of iodine deficiency disorders* (eds. B.S. Hetzel, J.T. Dunn, and J.B. Stanbury). Elsevier, Amsterdam.

World Health Organization (1986). *Report of the 39th World Health Assembly Resolution 29*, Geneva.

Index